I0841464

RADIANT AT 40 AND BEYOND

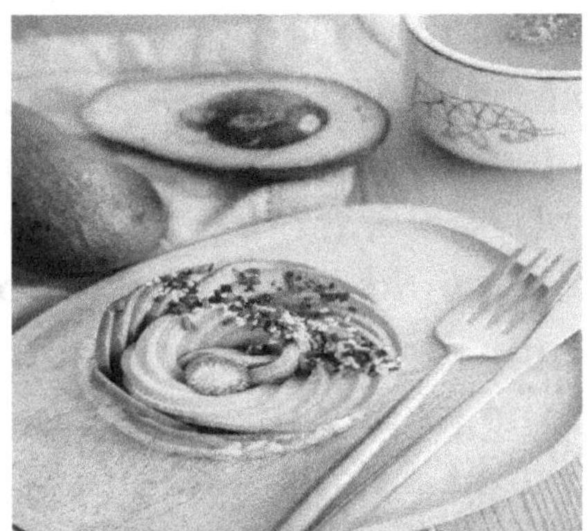

Your Essential Guide to a 14 Days Healthy Aging Diet: Boost immunity, promote longevity, lower inflammation, detoxify and lose weight.

BY

AURELIA GREY

Copyright © 2023 by Audrey Parker.

All rights reserved. No part of this publication may be reproduced, distributed, or transmitted in any form or by any means, including photocopying, recording, or other electronic or mechanical methods, without the prior written permission of the copyright holder, except in the case of brief quotations embodied in critical reviews and certain other noncommercial uses permitted by copyright law.

Table of Contents

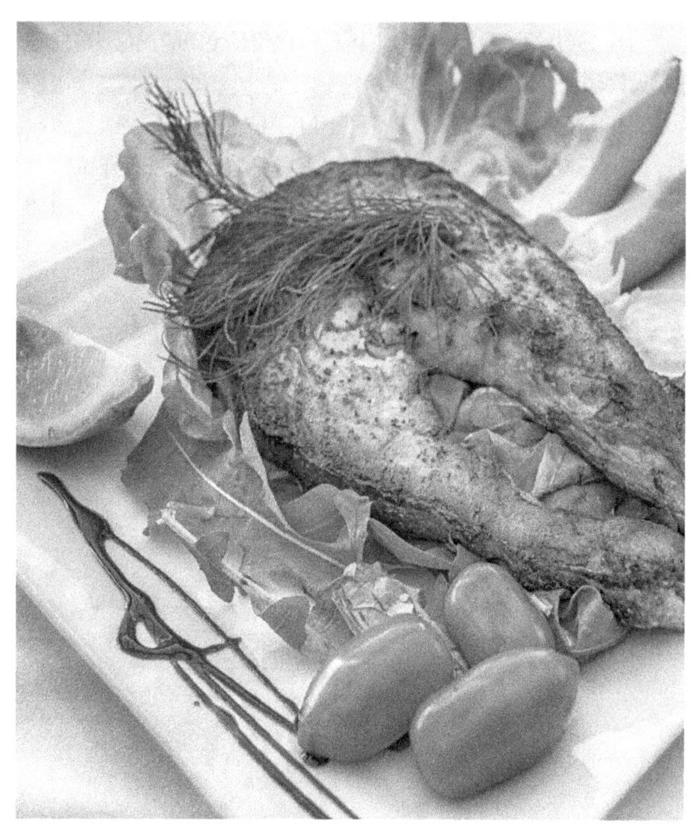

INTRODUCTION

The 14-day balanced diet for healthy aging aims to enhance various aspects of well-being for women over 40. It involves incorporating nutrient-dense foods that boost immunity, such as fruits and vegetables rich in vitamins and antioxidants. To promote longevity, the diet emphasizes whole grains, lean proteins, and healthy fats.

Lowering inflammation is addressed by including anti-inflammatory foods like fatty fish and nuts. Detoxification is encouraged through hydration and consumption of foods with detoxifying properties, such as cruciferous vegetables. Additionally, the plan supports weight loss by promoting a calorie-conscious, balanced approach to eating.

OVERVIEW OF HEALTHY AGING

The importance of healthy aging lies in maintaining physical, mental, and social well-being as individuals grow older. It involves adopting lifestyle choices and practices that enhance quality of life and longevity. Key aspects of the importance of healthy aging include:

1. Maintaining Independence: Healthy aging supports the ability to live independently, engage in daily activities, and maintain a good quality of life without undue reliance on others.
2. Preventing Disease and Disability: A focus on health can help prevent or manage chronic conditions associated with aging, reducing the risk of disease and disability.
3. Cognitive Function: Adopting a healthy lifestyle, including proper nutrition and regular exercise, contributes to cognitive health, potentially lowering the risk of cognitive decline and conditions like dementia.
4. Emotional Well-being: Healthy aging promotes emotional and mental well-being, fostering resilience and a positive outlook on life.
5. Social Connections: Staying socially active and maintaining relationships is

crucial for mental health and can contribute to a sense of purpose and belonging.
6. Physical Fitness: Regular exercise and a balanced diet support physical fitness, muscle strength, and flexibility, contributing to overall mobility and reducing the risk of falls.
7. Adaptability: Healthy aging involves adapting to life changes, such as retirement or lifestyle adjustments, with resilience and a proactive mindset.
8. Longevity with Quality of Life: The goal is not just to extend life but to increase the number of healthy, active years, promoting longevity with a high quality of life.
9. Nutritional Considerations: Recognizing the importance of a well-balanced diet rich in nutrients, vitamins, and minerals to address changing nutritional needs and support various bodily functions.

In summary, embracing the principles of healthy aging is essential for individuals to enjoy a fulfilling and active life throughout their later years.

IMPORTANCE OF BALANCED NUTRITION

Balanced nutrition involves consuming a variety of foods in appropriate quantities to provide the body with the essential nutrients it needs for optimal health. A balanced diet usually consists of a combination of:

Macronutrients:

- Carbohydrates: Found in grains, fruits, and vegetables, they are a primary source of energy.
- Proteins: Obtained from sources like meat, dairy, legumes, and nuts, they are essential for building and repairing tissues.
- Fats: Found in oils, nuts, and avocados, they are important for energy, nutrient absorption, and cell function.

2. Micronutrients:
    - Vitamins: Essential for various bodily functions, vitamins are found in fruits, vegetables, dairy, and other food sources.

     ○ Minerals: Critical for bone health, nerve function, and more, minerals are present in foods like leafy greens, dairy, and nuts.

3. Fiber:
     ○ Found in whole grains, fruits, and vegetables, fiber supports digestive health and helps maintain a feeling of fullness.

A balanced diet involves managing portion sizes, choosing a variety of nutrient-dense foods, and considering individual nutritional needs based on factors such as age, sex, activity level, and health status.

Key principles of balanced nutrition include moderation, variety, and proportionality. It aims to meet the body's energy needs while providing the necessary nutrients for overall well-being, disease prevention, and optimal functioning. Consulting with a healthcare professional or nutritionist can help tailor dietary recommendations to individual requirements.

Balanced nutrition is crucial for several reasons:

1. Optimal Health: A balanced diet provides the necessary nutrients— carbohydrates, proteins, fats, vitamins, and minerals—essential for the proper functioning of the body. This supports overall health and well-being.
2. Energy Production: Carbohydrates are a primary source of energy, and a balanced diet ensures an adequate supply for daily activities and bodily functions.
3. Metabolism Support: Proper nutrition supports a healthy metabolism, influencing how the body converts food into energy and how efficiently it uses that energy.
4. Disease Prevention: A balanced diet can help prevent chronic diseases by providing the nutrients that contribute to a strong immune system and overall cellular health.
5. Weight Management: Balanced nutrition promotes a healthy weight by providing nutrients in appropriate quantities,

preventing overconsumption of calories, and supporting metabolism.

6. Mental Health: Nutrient-rich foods contribute to cognitive function and emotional well-being. For example, omega-3 fatty acids found in fish are associated with brain health.
7. Digestive Health: A diet rich in fiber, obtained from fruits, vegetables, and whole grains, supports digestive health, preventing constipation and promoting a healthy gut microbiome.
8. Bone Health: To maintain strong bones and fend off diseases like osteoporosis, a sufficient diet rich in calcium and vitamin D is necessary.
9. Heart Health: Balanced nutrition, particularly a diet low in saturated fats and cholesterol, contributes to heart health by maintaining healthy blood pressure and cholesterol levels.
10. Long-Term Wellness: Adopting a balanced diet as a part of a sustainable and long-term lifestyle promotes overall wellness, helping individuals age with vitality and reducing the risk of nutritional deficiencies.

In summary, balanced nutrition is fundamental for supporting physical health, preventing diseases, managing weight, and promoting overall well-being across the lifespan.

CHAPTER 1

UNDERSTANDING THE AGING PROCESS

Understanding the aging process involves recognizing the complex and gradual changes that occur in the human body over time. Key aspects of the aging process include:

1. Metabolic Changes:
   - As individuals age, the metabolic rate tends to decline. This can result in a decrease in the number of calories the body burns at rest, influencing weight management.
2. Hormonal Influences:
   - Hormonal changes, particularly in women during menopause, can impact various bodily functions. For example, a decrease in estrogen levels can affect bone density and fat distribution.

3. Muscle Mass and Strength:
    o   There is a natural decline in muscle mass and strength with age. This can contribute to a reduction in overall physical activity and metabolism.
4. Bone Density:
    o   As people age, their bone density tends to decrease, increasing their risk of osteoporosis and fractures. It is essential to consume enough calcium and vitamin D to keep your bones healthy.
5. Cognitive Changes:
    o   Cognitive function may experience changes, including a potential decline in memory and processing speed. However, cognitive decline is not universal, and healthy lifestyle choices can positively influence brain health.
6. Skin Changes:
    o   The skin undergoes changes such as reduced elasticity, leading to wrinkles and sagging. Protection from sun exposure

and proper skincare become increasingly important.
7. Vision and Hearing:
     o Aging is often accompanied by changes in hearing and vision. Regular eye and ear check-ups become crucial for maintaining sensory health.
8. Immune System Function:
     o The immune system may weaken, making individuals more susceptible to infections and illnesses. Proper nutrition and healthy habits can support immune function.

Understanding these aspects of the aging process allows individuals to make informed lifestyle choices that can positively influence their health and well-being as they age. Adopting a proactive approach, including a balanced diet, regular exercise, and preventive healthcare measures, can contribute to healthy aging and an improved quality of life.

1. METABOLIC CHANGES

Metabolic changes refer to alterations in the body's metabolic rate and processes as part of the natural aging process. Several key metabolic changes occur with age:

1. Decreased Basal Metabolic Rate (BMR):
    - BMR, the number of calories the body needs at rest to maintain basic physiological functions, tends to decrease with age. This decline can contribute to weight gain if dietary habits are not adjusted accordingly.
2. Changes in Body Composition:
    - Aging is often associated with a shift in body composition, including a decrease in lean muscle mass and an increase in body fat. Since muscle tissue burns more calories than fat, this change can further impact metabolic rate.
3. Hormonal Influence:

- Hormonal changes, such as a decrease in growth hormone and sex hormones, can affect metabolism. For example, menopause in women is associated with a decline in estrogen, impacting both weight distribution and metabolic processes.

4. Insulin Sensitivity:
   - Insulin sensitivity may decrease with age, affecting the body's ability to regulate blood sugar levels. This can contribute to an increased risk of insulin resistance and type 2 diabetes.

5. Mitochondrial Function:
   - Mitochondria, the cellular structures responsible for energy production, may experience changes with age. Reduced mitochondrial function can impact the efficiency of energy conversion.

6. Physical Activity Levels:
   - As individuals age, there may be a tendency to become less physically active. A sedentary

lifestyle can further contribute to a decline in metabolic rate and muscle mass.

Understanding these metabolic changes is essential for adopting lifestyle practices that support healthy aging. Strategies such as regular physical activity, a balanced diet, and resistance training can help mitigate the impact of metabolic changes, promoting overall well-being and weight management.

HORMONAL INFLUENCES ESPECIALLY DURING MENOPAUSE

Hormonal influences, particularly during menopause, play a significant role in shaping various aspects of a woman's health. Menopause typically occurs between the ages of 45 and 55, marking the end of the reproductive years. Key hormonal changes during menopause include:

1. Estrogen Decline:

- Menopause involves a natural decline in estrogen levels. Estrogen plays a crucial role in regulating the menstrual cycle and has various effects on the body, including maintaining bone density and supporting heart health.

2. Progesterone Changes:
   - Progesterone, another reproductive hormone, also decreases during menopause. This hormone is involved in regulating the menstrual cycle and supporting pregnancy.

3. Impact on Bone Health:
   - The decline in estrogen levels can lead to a reduction in bone density, increasing the risk of osteoporosis. Adequate calcium and vitamin D intake, along with weight-bearing exercise, become essential for maintaining bone health.

4. Vasomotor Symptoms:
   - Hormonal fluctuations during menopause can contribute to vasomotor symptoms, such as

hot flashes and night sweats. While these symptoms are temporary, they can significantly affect a woman's quality of life.

5. Changes in Fat Distribution:
    - Estrogen influences the distribution of body fat, and its decline during menopause can result in an increase in abdominal fat. This shift in fat distribution is associated with an increased risk of cardiovascular disease.
6. Impact on Mood and Mental Health:
    - Hormonal changes during menopause can influence mood and mental health. Some women may experience mood swings, irritability, or an increased risk of depression during this transition.

Understanding these hormonal influences is crucial for women going through menopause and for healthcare professionals providing support and guidance. Lifestyle adjustments, including a balanced diet, regular exercise, and stress management, can help alleviate some of the challenges associated with hormonal changes during this stage of life.

IMPACT IN MUSCLE MASS AND WEIGHT DISTRIBUTION

The impact on muscle mass and weight distribution is a notable aspect of hormonal changes, especially during menopause. Several factors contribute to these changes:

1. Muscle Mass Decline:
   - With age and hormonal shifts, there is a natural decline in muscle mass, a condition known as sarcopenia. Reduced estrogen levels during menopause may accelerate this process. Loss of muscle mass can influence metabolism and decrease overall strength.
2. Increase in Body Fat:
   - Hormonal changes, particularly the decline in estrogen, are associated with an increase in body fat, especially around the abdomen. This shift in fat distribution contributes to

changes in overall body
composition.

3. Metabolic Impact:
    - Compared to fat tissue, muscle
      tissue burns more calories when
      at rest because it has a higher
      metabolic activity. The decline in
      muscle mass can result in a
      slower metabolism, making it
      easier to gain weight and
      potentially more challenging to
      lose weight.

4. Influence on Physical Activity:
    - Changes in hormonal levels and
      body composition can impact
      energy levels and motivation for
      physical activity. Maintaining or
      increasing physical activity,
      including strength training
      exercises, becomes crucial for
      preserving muscle mass and
      managing weight.

5. Bone Health Connection:
    - The decline in estrogen not only
      affects muscle mass but also
      impacts bone density. Weight-
      bearing exercises that support
      muscle strength also contribute to

maintaining bone health during menopause.

6. Strategies for Weight Management:
    - Adopting a balanced diet, rich in nutrients, and engaging in regular exercise, including both aerobic and resistance training, can help mitigate the effects of hormonal changes. These lifestyle strategies support muscle maintenance, boost metabolism, and aid in weight management.

Understanding and addressing the impact on muscle mass and weight distribution during hormonal changes, such as menopause, involves a holistic approach that combines proper nutrition, regular exercise, and overall lifestyle modifications.

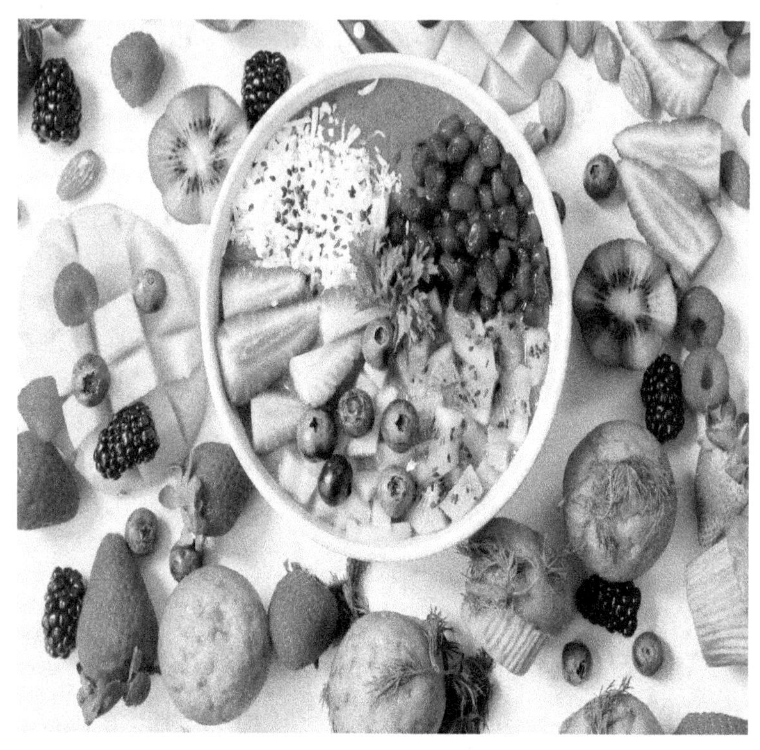

CHAPTER 2

PRINCIPLES OF THE 14-DAY BALANCED DIET

The principles of the 14-day balanced diet focus on providing essential nutrients while addressing specific goals like boosting immunity, promoting longevity, lowering inflammation, supporting detoxification, and facilitating weight loss for women over 40. Here are key principles:

1. Nutrient-Dense Foods:
    - Prioritize whole, minimally processed foods rich in nutrients, including fruits, vegetables, lean proteins, whole grains, and healthy fats.
2. Lean Proteins:
    - Incorporate lean protein sources such as poultry, fish, legumes, and tofu to support muscle health

and provide essential amino acids.

3. Whole Grains:
    - Choose whole grains like brown rice, quinoa, and oats for complex carbohydrates, fiber, and sustained energy.
4. Fruits and Vegetables:
    - Include a variety of colorful fruits and vegetables to provide vitamins, minerals, antioxidants, and fiber.
5. Healthy Fats:
    - Incorporate sources of healthy fats, such as avocados, nuts, seeds, and olive oil, for heart health and satiety.
6. Immunity-Boosting Components:
    - Include foods rich in antioxidants, vitamins (especially C and E), and minerals to support the immune system.
7. Anti-Inflammatory Foods:
    - Choose foods with anti-inflammatory properties, including fatty fish, turmeric, ginger, and leafy greens, to help lower inflammation.

8. Hydration:
    o Stay well-hydrated by drinking water throughout the day. Hydration supports overall health, digestion, and detoxification.
9. Detoxification Support:
    o Include foods that support natural detoxification processes, such as cruciferous vegetables, and promote liver health.
10. Calorie Consciousness:
    o Be mindful of portion sizes and overall calorie intake to support weight management goals.
11. Balanced Approach:
    o Aim for a balanced distribution of macronutrients (carbohydrates, proteins, fats) to meet energy needs and maintain overall balance.
12. Variety and Moderation:
    o Embrace a variety of foods and avoid extremes. Enjoy treats in moderation while maintaining a focus on nutrient-rich choices.
13. Meal Timing:
    o Consider the timing of meals to support energy levels throughout

the day and avoid prolonged
periods of hunger.

14. Adaptability:
   - Recognize that nutritional needs may vary, and the diet can be adapted based on individual preferences, health conditions, and goals.

These principles provide a foundation for a well-rounded and sustainable approach to nutrition, fostering overall health and well-being during the 14-day balanced diet.

NUTRIENT-DENSE FOODS

Meals that are high in essential nutrients in relation to their calorie content are considered nutrient-dense. These foods offer a wealth of vitamins, minerals, antioxidants, and other beneficial compounds. Here are examples of nutrient-dense foods:

1. Leafy Greens:

- Spinach, kale, Swiss chard, and other dark leafy greens are rich in vitamins A, C, K, and minerals like iron and calcium.
2. Berries:
   - Blueberries, strawberries, raspberries, and blackberries are packed with antioxidants, fiber, and vitamins.
3. Cruciferous Vegetables:
   - Broccoli, cauliflower, Brussels sprouts, and cabbage provide fiber, vitamins, and compounds with potential anti-cancer properties.
4. Colorful Vegetables:
   - Bell peppers, carrots, sweet potatoes, and tomatoes offer a variety of vitamins, minerals, and antioxidants.
5. Fruits:
   - Apples, oranges, bananas, and other fruits are nutrient-dense, providing essential vitamins, fiber, and natural sugars.
6. Lean Proteins:
   - Chicken, turkey, fish, tofu, and legumes are excellent sources of

protein, essential amino acids, and various minerals.

7. Nuts and Seeds:
    - Almonds, walnuts, chia seeds, and flaxseeds are rich in healthy fats, protein, fiber, and essential nutrients.
8. Whole Grains:
    - Quinoa, brown rice, oats, and whole wheat provide complex carbohydrates, fiber, and essential minerals.
9. Fatty Fish:
    - Salmon, mackerel, and sardines are high in omega-3 fatty acids, which support heart and brain health.
10. Dairy or Dairy Alternatives:
    - Greek yogurt, milk, and fortified plant-based alternatives offer calcium, vitamin D, and protein.
11. Eggs:
    - Eggs are a nutrient-dense source of protein, vitamins, and minerals, including B-vitamins and choline.
12. Legumes:
    - Beans, lentils, and chickpeas provide plant-based protein, fiber,

and a variety of vitamins and minerals.

13. Lean Meats:
    - Lean cuts of beef or pork contain protein, iron, zinc, and other essential nutrients.
14. Tomatoes:
    - Tomatoes are rich in antioxidants, particularly lycopene, which is associated with various health benefits.

Including a variety of these nutrient-dense foods in your diet supports overall health, helps meet nutritional needs, and can contribute to weight management and disease prevention.

LEAN PROTEINS

Lean proteins are excellent sources of high-quality protein with relatively low fat content. Incorporating lean proteins into your diet is beneficial for muscle health, weight management, and overall well-being. Here are some examples of lean proteins:

1. Chicken Breast:
    - Skinless, boneless chicken breast is a lean source of protein that can be grilled, baked, or sautéed.
2. Turkey:
    - Lean ground turkey or skinless turkey breast provides protein with less fat. It works well in a variety of recipes and is adaptable.
3. Fish:
    - Omega-3 fatty acids are abundant in fatty fish, such as salmon, trout, and mackerel. Other lean fish options include cod, haddock, and tilapia.
4. Seafood:
    - Shrimp, scallops, and other shellfish are low in fat and high in protein. They also provide essential minerals like zinc and selenium.
5. Lean Cuts of Beef:
    - Choose lean cuts such as sirloin, tenderloin, or round steaks. Trim visible fat before cooking to keep them lean.

6. Pork Tenderloin:
   - Pork tenderloin is a lean cut that can be roasted, grilled, or stir-fried. Trimming visible fat helps reduce its overall fat content.
7. Lean Ground Meat:
   - Opt for lean ground meats such as lean ground beef (90% lean or higher) or ground turkey (lean or extra lean) for a variety of recipes.
8. Chicken Thighs (Skinless):
   - While chicken thighs have slightly more fat than breast meat, choosing skinless thighs can still provide a good source of protein.
9. Greek Yogurt:
   - Greek yogurt is higher in protein compared to regular yogurt and can be a versatile addition to meals or snacks.
10. Cottage Cheese:
   - Cottage cheese is a dairy product that is rich in protein and can be included in both sweet and savory dishes.
11. Eggs:

- o Eggs are an affordable and versatile source of protein. Opt for egg whites if you're looking to minimize fat intake.

12. Tofu:
    - o One low-fat plant-based source of protein is tofu. It works well in recipes that are sweet or savory.

Incorporating a variety of lean proteins into your diet helps ensure a balanced intake of essential amino acids while promoting heart health and weight management.

WHOLE GRAINS

Whole grains are grains that contain the entire grain kernel – the bran, germ, and endosperm. Unlike refined grains, which are processed to remove the bran and germ, whole grains retain their nutritional integrity, providing essential nutrients, fiber, and other health benefits. These are a few instances of whole grains:

1. Quinoa:
   - A versatile grain rich in protein, fiber, and various vitamins and minerals.
2. Brown Rice:
   - A whole grain with a nutty flavor, brown rice is a good source of fiber, B-vitamins, and minerals.
3. Oats:
   - Oats are high in soluble fiber and provide beta-glucans, known for their heart health benefits.
4. Barley:
   - Barley is rich in fiber, vitamins, and minerals. It can be used in soups, stews, or as a side dish.
5. Buckwheat:
   - Buckwheat, despite its name, is gluten-free and not related to wheat. It offers protein, fiber, and various antioxidants.
6. Quinoa:
   - A complete protein source, quinoa is gluten-free and provides a good balance of amino acids.
7. Farro:

o An ancient grain with a chewy texture, farro contains fiber, protein, and nutrients like magnesium and iron.

8. Whole Wheat:
    o Products made from 100% whole wheat flour, such as whole wheat bread or pasta, retain the nutritional benefits of the entire grain.

9. Millet:
    o Millet is a gluten-free grain rich in antioxidants, magnesium, and other essential nutrients.

10. Amaranth:
    o Amaranth is a gluten-free grain high in protein, fiber, and various vitamins and minerals.

11. Freekeh:
    o An ancient grain made from roasted green wheat, freekeh is high in protein, fiber, and minerals.

12. Sorghum:
    o A gluten-free grain that is rich in antioxidants, fiber, and various nutrients.

Including a variety of whole grains in your diet supports digestive health, provides sustained energy, and offers a range of essential nutrients. When choosing whole grain products, look for items labeled "100% whole grain" to ensure you're getting the full nutritional benefits.

FRUITS AND VEGETABLES

Fruits and vegetables are essential components of a balanced and nutritious diet, providing a wide range of vitamins, minerals, fiber, and antioxidants. Including a variety of colorful fruits and vegetables in your meals supports overall health and helps prevent chronic diseases. Here are examples of fruits and vegetables to incorporate into your diet:

Fruits:

1. Berries:
    - Blackberries, raspberries, strawberries, and blueberries are high in vitamins and antioxidants.

2. Citrus Fruits:
   - Oranges, grapefruits, lemons, and limes provide vitamin C, fiber, and various other nutrients.
3. Apples:
   - Apples are a good source of fiber and contain antioxidants, including flavonoids.
4. Bananas:
   - Bananas are rich in potassium, vitamin B6, and provide a quick source of energy.
5. Kiwi:
   - Kiwi is a great source of dietary fiber, vitamin K, and vitamin C.
6. Avocado:
   - Avocado is a nutrient-dense fruit high in healthy monounsaturated fats, potassium, and vitamins.
7. Mango:
   - Mangoes are rich in vitamin C, vitamin A, and provide natural sweetness.
8. Pineapple:
   - Pineapple contains bromelain, an enzyme with potential anti-inflammatory benefits, and is a good source of vitamin C.

9. Grapes:
    - Grapes, particularly red grapes, contain antioxidants like resveratrol.
10. Pears:
    - Pears offer dietary fiber, vitamins, and minerals.

Vegetables:

1. Leafy Greens:
    - Spinach, kale, Swiss chard, and collard greens are nutrient-dense leafy vegetables.
2. Broccoli:
    - Broccoli is rich in vitamins C and K, fiber, and various antioxidants.
3. Carrots:
    - Vitamin A is produced by the body from beta-carotene, which is found in carrots.
4. Bell Peppers:
    - Bell peppers are high in vitamin C and contain antioxidants.
5. Tomatoes:

- A powerful antioxidant with several health advantages, lycopene is abundant in tomatoes.

6. Cauliflower:
   - Cauliflower is a versatile vegetable that provides fiber, vitamins, and minerals.
7. Sweet Potatoes:
   - Sweet potatoes are rich in beta-carotene, vitamins, and fiber.
8. Zucchini:
   - Zucchini is a low-calorie vegetable rich in vitamins and minerals.
9. Brussels Sprouts:
   - Brussels sprouts are high in fiber, vitamin C, and vitamin K.
10. Cabbage:
    - Cabbage is a cruciferous vegetable with potential health benefits.

Incorporating a colorful array of fruits and vegetables into your meals ensures a diverse range of nutrients, promoting overall health and well-being.

HEALTHY FATS

Healthy fats are an essential part of a balanced diet and play a crucial role in supporting overall health. These fats provide necessary fatty acids, aid in nutrient absorption, and contribute to various bodily functions. Here are examples of healthy fats to include in your diet:

1. Avocados:
    - Avocados are rich in monounsaturated fats, which are heart-healthy and contribute to a feeling of satiety.
2. Olive Oil:
    - Extra virgin olive oil is a source of monounsaturated fats and contains antioxidants with potential anti-inflammatory benefits.
3. Nuts:
    - Almonds, walnuts, pistachios, and other nuts provide monounsaturated and

polyunsaturated fats, along with fiber, vitamins, and minerals.

4. Seeds:
    - Chia seeds, flaxseeds, sunflower seeds, and pumpkin seeds are good sources of omega-3 fatty acids, fiber, and various nutrients.
5. Fatty Fish:
    - Salmon, mackerel, trout, and sardines are rich in omega-3 fatty acids, supporting heart and brain health.
6. Coconut Oil:
    - Coconut oil contains saturated fats, but they are mostly in the form of medium-chain triglycerides (MCTs), which may have metabolic benefits.
7. Fatty Fish:
    - Salmon, mackerel, trout, and sardines are rich in omega-3 fatty acids, supporting heart and brain health.
8. Flaxseed Oil:
    - Flaxseed oil is a plant-based source of omega-3 fatty acids.
9. Chia Seeds:

- ○ Chia seeds are high in omega-3 fatty acids, fiber, and various nutrients.
10. Dark Chocolate:
   - ○ Dark chocolate in moderation provides monounsaturated fats and antioxidants.
11. Nut Butters:
   - ○ Natural peanut butter, almond butter, or other nut butters offer healthy fats and protein.
12. Cheese:
   - ○ Some types of cheese, like feta or goat cheese, contain healthy fats along with calcium and protein.
13. Eggs:
   - ○ Eggs, especially those enriched with omega-3 fatty acids, provide a source of healthy fats.
14. Soybeans and Tofu:
   - ○ Soy-based products like tofu and edamame contain polyunsaturated fats and are good plant-based protein sources.

Incorporating these healthy fats into your diet supports various bodily functions, including brain health, hormone production, and the absorption of fat-soluble vitamins. Remember to consume fats in moderation as part of a well-balanced diet.

IMMUNITY-BOOSTING COMPONENTS

Certain nutrients and compounds are known for their potential to boost the immune system. While no single food or supplement can guarantee immunity, including a variety of these components in your diet can support overall immune health. Here are key immunity-boosting components and examples of foods that contain them:

1. Vitamin C:
    - Found in citrus fruits (oranges, grapefruits), strawberries, kiwi, bell peppers, and broccoli. The function of immune cells depends on vitamin C.
2. Zinc:

a. Present in foods like lean meats, poultry, seafood, nuts, seeds, and legumes. Zinc is involved in immune cell function and wound healing.

3. Probiotics:
   a. present in fermented foods such as kimchi, kefir, yogurt, and sauerkraut. Probiotics support a healthy gut microbiome, influencing immune function.

4. Beta-Glucans:
   a. Found in oats, barley, mushrooms, and certain grains. Beta-glucans have immune-modulating properties.

5. Antioxidants:
   a. Present in a variety of fruits and vegetables, such as berries, spinach, kale, and tomatoes. Antioxidants help combat oxidative stress, supporting overall health.

6. Elderberry:
   a. Elderberries contain compounds with potential antiviral and immune-boosting properties.

7. Garlic:

a. Garlic has antimicrobial and immune-modulating effects. Include it in your diet for added flavor and potential health benefits.

8. Echinacea:
    a. Often used in herbal teas and supplements, echinacea may have immune-enhancing properties.

9. Turmeric:
    a. Contains curcumin, which has anti-inflammatory and antioxidant effects. Add turmeric to dishes or enjoy it in teas.

10. Ginger:
    a. Ginger has anti-inflammatory and antioxidant properties. Use fresh ginger in cooking or enjoy it in teas.

11. Green Tea:
    a. Green tea is rich in antioxidants, including catechins, which may have immune-boosting effects.

12. Citrus Bioflavonoids:
    a. Present in citrus fruits, these compounds have antioxidant and anti-inflammatory properties.

13. Omega-3 Fatty Acids:
    a. found in walnuts, flaxseeds, chia seeds, and fatty fish (salmon, mackerel). Found in walnuts, flaxseeds, chia seeds, and fatty fish (salmon, mackerel). Omega-3s support immune cell function and reduce inflammation.

Remember that a well-balanced diet, along with other healthy lifestyle practices like regular exercise, adequate sleep, and stress management, contributes to a robust immune system.

ANTIOXIDANT-RICH FOODS

Antioxidant-rich foods help combat oxidative stress in the body, which is associated with various chronic diseases and aging. Including a variety of these foods in your diet supports overall health and well-being. Here are examples of antioxidant-rich foods:

1. Berries:
   - Blueberries, strawberries, raspberries, and blackberries are packed with antioxidants like anthocyanins and vitamin C.
2. Dark Chocolate:
   - Dark chocolate contains flavonoids, which have antioxidant properties. Choose chocolate with higher cocoa content for more antioxidants.
3. Artichokes:
   - Artichokes are a good source of antioxidants, including quercetin, which may have anti-inflammatory effects.
4. Nuts:
   - Almonds, walnuts, and pistachios provide vitamin E, selenium, and other antioxidants.
5. Spinach:
   - Spinach is rich in various antioxidants, including lutein and zeaxanthin.
6. Kale:
   - Kale contains antioxidants like beta-carotene, lutein, and vitamin C.

7. Broccoli:
   - Broccoli is a cruciferous vegetable rich in antioxidants, including sulforaphane.
8. Tomatoes:
   - Tomatoes contain lycopene, a powerful antioxidant associated with various health benefits.
9. Red and Yellow Bell Peppers:
   - These peppers provide vitamin C and other antioxidants that support immune health.
10. Carrots:
    - Carrots are high in beta-carotene, an antioxidant that the body converts into vitamin A.
11. Sweet Potatoes:
    - Sweet potatoes contain beta-carotene, vitamins, and minerals with antioxidant properties.
12. Oranges and Citrus Fruits:
    - Citrus fruits provide vitamin C, a potent antioxidant that supports immune function.
13. Green Tea:
    - Green tea contains catechins, which are antioxidants with potential health benefits.

14. Turmeric:
    - Turmeric contains curcumin, an antioxidant with anti-inflammatory properties.
15. Grapes:
    - Grapes, especially red and purple varieties, contain resveratrol, an antioxidant associated with heart health.
16. Avocado:
    - Avocado provides vitamin E and other antioxidants along with healthy monounsaturated fats.
17. Cranberries:
    - Cranberries are rich in antioxidants, particularly anthocyanins.
18. Pomegranate:
    - Pomegranate seeds and juice contain antioxidants like punicalagins and anthocyanins.

Including a variety of these antioxidant-rich foods in your diet helps promote overall health, protect cells from damage, and may contribute to disease prevention.

VITAMINS AND MINERALS

Vitamins and minerals are essential micronutrients that play crucial roles in various physiological functions, supporting overall health and well-being. Here's an overview of important vitamins and minerals and the foods where you can find them:

Vitamins:

1. Vitamin A:
   - Sources: Carrots, sweet potatoes, spinach, kale, eggs, and liver.
   - Functions: Important for vision, immune function, and skin health.
2. Vitamin B Complex:
   - Includes B1 (Thiamine), B2 (Riboflavin), B3 (Niacin), B5 (Pantothenic Acid), B6 (Pyridoxine), B7 (Biotin), B9 (Folate), B12 (Cobalamin).

- Sources: Whole grains, nuts, seeds, meat, poultry, fish, dairy, leafy greens.
- Functions: Support energy metabolism, nervous system health, and red blood cell formation.

3. Vitamin C:
- Sources: Citrus fruits (oranges, lemons), strawberries, bell peppers, broccoli.
- Functions: Antioxidant, supports immune function, aids in collagen synthesis.

4. Vitamin D:
- Sources: Sunlight, fatty fish (salmon, mackerel), fortified dairy products.
- Functions: Facilitates calcium absorption, supports bone health and immune function.

5. Vitamin E:
- Sources: Nuts, seeds, spinach, broccoli, sunflower oil.
- Functions: Antioxidant, supports skin health, and protects cell membranes.

6. Vitamin K:

- Sources: Leafy greens (kale, spinach, broccoli), Brussels sprouts.
  - Functions: Essential for blood clotting and bone health.

Minerals:

1. Calcium:
   - Sources: Dairy products, leafy greens (kale, collard greens), almonds, fortified foods.
   - Functions: Critical for bone health, nerve transmission, and muscle function.
2. Iron:
   - Sources: Red meat, poultry, fish, lentils, beans, fortified cereals.
   - Functions: Essential for oxygen transport in the blood (hemoglobin).
3. Magnesium:
   - Sources: Nuts, seeds, whole grains, leafy greens, beans.

- Functions: Supports muscle and nerve function, bone health, and energy metabolism.

4. Potassium:
   - Sources: Bananas, oranges, potatoes, spinach, beans.
   - Functions: Regulates fluid balance, supports nerve transmission and muscle function.

5. Zinc:
   - Sources: Meat, poultry, dairy products, beans, nuts, seeds.
   - Functions: Supports immune function, wound healing, and DNA synthesis.

6. Selenium:
   - Sources: Brazil nuts, fish, poultry, whole grains, eggs.
   - Functions: Antioxidant, supports thyroid function.

7. Iodine:
   - Sources: Seafood, iodized salt, dairy products.
   - Functions: Essential for thyroid hormone production.

8. Copper:

- Sources: Shellfish, nuts, seeds, beans, whole grains.
- Functions: Supports iron metabolism, collagen formation.

Ensuring a well-balanced diet that includes a variety of nutrient-rich foods helps meet your body's vitamin and mineral needs.

INFLAMMATIONS-LOWERING STRATEGIES

Reducing inflammation in the body is important for overall health and may help prevent or manage various chronic conditions. Here are strategies to help lower inflammation:

1. Anti-Inflammatory Diet:
   - Focus on whole, unprocessed foods such as fruits, vegetables, whole grains, lean proteins, and healthy fats. Minimize processed foods, sugary drinks, and excessive consumption of red and processed meats.

2. Omega-3 Fatty Acids:
    - Include fatty fish (salmon, mackerel, sardines), flaxseeds, chia seeds, and walnuts in your diet. Omega-3 fatty acids have anti-inflammatory properties.
3. Colorful Fruits and Vegetables:
    - Consume a variety of colorful fruits and vegetables rich in antioxidants, vitamins, and minerals. These can help combat oxidative stress and reduce inflammation.
4. Turmeric and Ginger:
    - Incorporate turmeric and ginger into your diet. These spices contain compounds with anti-inflammatory and antioxidant effects.
5. Extra Virgin Olive Oil:
    - Use extra virgin olive oil as your primary cooking oil. It contains monounsaturated fats and compounds that may have anti-inflammatory properties.
6. Nuts and Seeds:
    - Include nuts (almonds, walnuts) and seeds (flaxseeds, chia

seeds) in your diet. They provide healthy fats and anti-inflammatory compounds.

7. Whole Grains:
    - Choose whole grains like brown rice, quinoa, and oats over refined grains. Whole grains contain fiber and other nutrients that may help reduce inflammation.
8. Probiotics:
    - Consume probiotic-rich foods like yogurt, kefir, and sauerkraut. Probiotics support gut health, influencing inflammation and immune function.
9. Green Tea:
    - Drink green tea regularly. It contains polyphenols with anti-inflammatory and antioxidant properties.
10. Hydration:
    - Stay well-hydrated by drinking plenty of water. Proper hydration supports overall health and helps flush out toxins.
11. Regular Exercise:

- Engage in regular physical activity. Exercise can have anti-inflammatory effects and contribute to overall well-being.

12. Adequate Sleep:
    - Ensure you get enough quality sleep. Sleep is crucial for the body's natural healing processes and can impact inflammation levels.

13. Stress Management:
    - Practice stress-reducing activities such as meditation, deep breathing exercises, or yoga. Chronic stress can contribute to inflammation.

14. Limit Alcohol Intake:
    - Consume alcohol in moderation. Excessive alcohol intake can contribute to inflammation.

15. Avoid Smoking:
    - If you smoke, consider quitting. Smoking is associated with increased inflammation and various health risks.

ANTI-INFLAMMATORY FOODS

Anti-inflammatory foods can help reduce inflammation in the body and promote overall health. Here are some foods known for their anti-inflammatory properties:

1. Fatty Fish:
   - Salmon, mackerel, sardines, and other fatty fish are rich in omega-3 fatty acids, which have potent anti-inflammatory effects.
2. Berries:
   - Blueberries, strawberries, raspberries, and blackberries are loaded with antioxidants and may help reduce inflammation.
3. Leafy Greens:
   - Spinach, kale, and other leafy greens contain vitamins, minerals, and antioxidants that combat inflammation.
4. Turmeric:
   - Curcumin, the active compound in turmeric, has strong anti-inflammatory and antioxidant properties.

5. Broccoli:
   - Broccoli is rich in sulforaphane, a compound with anti-inflammatory effects.
6. Avocado:
   - Avocados contain monounsaturated fats and antioxidants, contributing to their anti-inflammatory properties.
7. Walnuts:
   - Walnuts are a good source of omega-3 fatty acids and antioxidants, providing anti-inflammatory benefits.
8. Cherries:
   - Cherries, especially tart cherries, contain compounds that may help reduce inflammation and muscle soreness.
9. Ginger:
   - Ginger has anti-inflammatory and antioxidant properties and can be included in both sweet and savory dishes.
10. Green Tea:
   - Green tea contains polyphenols with anti-inflammatory and antioxidant effects.

11. Olive Oil:
   - Extra virgin olive oil is rich in monounsaturated fats and contains compounds that may reduce inflammation.
12. Tomatoes:
   - Tomatoes contain lycopene, an antioxidant with anti-inflammatory properties.
13. Dark Chocolate:
   - Dark chocolate with high cocoa content contains flavonoids that may have anti-inflammatory effects.
14. Pineapple:
   - Pineapple contains bromelain, an enzyme with potential anti-inflammatory benefits.
15. Bell Peppers:
   - Bell peppers are rich in antioxidants, including quercetin, which may have anti-inflammatory effects.
16. Garlic:
   - Garlic has anti-inflammatory and immune-boosting properties.
17. Nuts:

- 　o　Almonds, Brazil nuts, and other nuts provide healthy fats and antioxidants with anti-inflammatory effects.
18. Mushrooms:
    - o　Certain mushrooms, like shiitake and maitake, contain compounds that may modulate the immune system and have anti-inflammatory effects.

Including a variety of these anti-inflammatory foods in your diet can contribute to overall well-being and help manage inflammation. It's important to adopt a balanced and varied approach to nutrition for optimal health benefits.

HYDRATION IMPORTANCE

Staying hydrated is essential for preserving general health and wellbeing. These are some major justifications for why it's crucial to stay hydrated:

1. Cellular Function:

- o Water is essential for various cellular processes, including nutrient transport, temperature regulation, and waste elimination.

2. Temperature Regulation:
   - o Adequate hydration helps regulate body temperature through processes like sweating and respiration.
3. Joint Lubrication:
   - o Water provides lubrication to joints, promoting smooth movement and reducing the risk of joint discomfort.
4. Nutrient Transport:
   - o Water plays a vital role in transporting nutrients throughout the body, facilitating the absorption and distribution of essential substances.
5. Digestive Health:
   - o Proper hydration supports digestive processes, aiding in the breakdown and absorption of food. It helps prevent constipation and supports overall gastrointestinal health.
6. Cognitive Function:

- Dehydration can impair cognitive function, affecting concentration, alertness, and overall mental performance.
7. Energy Levels:
   - Staying hydrated helps maintain energy levels. Dehydration can lead to feelings of fatigue and reduced physical performance.
8. Kidney Function:
   - Adequate water intake is essential for proper kidney function, helping to flush out waste products and toxins from the body.
9. Skin Health:
   - Hydration contributes to skin elasticity and helps maintain a healthy complexion. Dehydration can lead to dry skin and an increased risk of skin issues.
10. Weight Management:
    - Drinking water before meals may contribute to a feeling of fullness, potentially supporting weight management by reducing calorie intake.
11. Exercise Performance:

- o Proper hydration is crucial for optimal athletic performance. Dehydration can lead to muscle cramps, fatigue, and impaired endurance.
12. Immune Function:
    - o Water is involved in the production and circulation of lymph, which plays a key role in the immune system.
13. Detoxification:
    - o Hydration supports the body's natural detoxification processes, aiding in the elimination of waste products.
14. Heart Health:
    - o Maintaining proper fluid balance is important for cardiovascular health, helping to regulate blood pressure and reduce the workload on the heart.
15. Prevention of Dehydration:
    - o Dehydration can have serious health consequences, ranging from mild symptoms like headache and dizziness to severe conditions such as heat-related illnesses.

To stay adequately hydrated, it's generally recommended to drink water throughout the day, adjusting intake based on individual factors such as age, activity level, and climate. While water is the primary source of hydration, other beverages and water-rich foods also contribute to overall fluid intake. It's important to pay attention to thirst cues and prioritize hydration for optimal health.

CHAPTER 3

DETOXIFICATION FOR HEALTHY AGING

The term "detoxification" describes how the body naturally gets rid of or balances out toxins. While the body has its built-in detoxification systems, there are lifestyle choices that can support these processes and contribute to healthy aging. Here are some strategies for promoting detoxification and overall well-being:

1. Hydration:
    - Adequate water intake is essential for flushing out toxins through urine and supporting various bodily functions. Try to have eight glasses of water or more each day.
2. Balanced Nutrition:
    - Consume a nutrient-dense, whole-foods-based diet rich in fruits, vegetables, whole grains, lean proteins, and healthy fats.

These foods provide essential nutrients that support the body's detoxification pathways.

3. Fiber-Rich Foods:
   - Consume fruits, vegetables, whole grains, and legumes to increase your intake of fiber. Fiber helps support digestive health and promotes regular bowel movements, aiding in the elimination of waste products.
4. Antioxidant-Rich Foods:
   - Eat foods high in antioxidants, such as berries, leafy greens, and other colorful fruits and vegetables. Antioxidants shield cells from harm and aid in the fight against oxidative stress.
5. Limit Processed Foods:
   - Minimize the intake of processed foods, which may contain additives, preservatives, and artificial ingredients. Choose whole, minimally processed foods to reduce exposure to potentially harmful substances.
6. Supportive Herbs and Spices:

- Incorporate herbs and spices with potential detoxifying properties into your diet. Examples include turmeric, ginger, cilantro, and parsley.

7. Exercise:
   - Engage in regular physical activity to support circulation, lymphatic flow, and sweat, all of which contribute to the elimination of toxins. Strength training and aerobic exercise have advantages.

8. Sauna or Steam Room:
   - Heat therapy through saunas or steam rooms may promote sweating, helping to eliminate toxins through the skin.

9. Adequate Sleep:
   - Prioritize quality sleep, as it is crucial for the body's natural repair and detoxification processes.

10. Limit Alcohol and Caffeine:
    - Moderation is key when consuming alcohol and caffeine. Excessive intake can burden the

liver, a key organ involved in detoxification.

11. Manage Stress:
    - Chronic stress can negatively impact overall health. Include stress-reduction methods in your routine, such as yoga, deep breathing, or meditation.

12. Liver Supportive Foods:
    - Include foods that support liver health, such as cruciferous vegetables (broccoli, cauliflower), beets, and garlic.

13. Intermittent Fasting:
    - Some studies suggest that intermittent fasting may support cellular repair and detoxification.

14. Limit Environmental Toxins:
    - Be mindful of your environment and try to reduce exposure to pollutants and toxins. This may include using natural cleaning products, choosing organic foods when possible, and being cautious with personal care products.

It's essential to note that extreme or prolonged detox diets may not be necessary or beneficial. The body's natural detoxification systems generally function well when supported by a healthy lifestyle.

FOODS SUPPORTING DETOX

Certain foods are known for their potential to support the body's natural detoxification processes. Including these foods in your diet can contribute to overall well-being. Here are some foods that may support detoxification:

1. Cruciferous Vegetables:
   - Broccoli, cauliflower, Brussels sprouts, and kale contain compounds that support liver detoxification enzymes.
2. Leafy Greens:
   - Spinach, kale, chard, and other leafy greens provide chlorophyll, which may support detoxification and help neutralize toxins.
3. Berries:

- Blueberries, strawberries, raspberries, and blackberries are rich in antioxidants, supporting the body's defense against oxidative stress.

4. Citrus Fruits:
   - Lemons, limes, oranges, and grapefruits contain vitamin C and other compounds that support liver detoxification.

5. Turmeric:
   - Curcumin, the active compound in turmeric, has anti-inflammatory and antioxidant properties that may support detoxification.

6. Ginger:
   - Ginger has anti-inflammatory effects and may support digestive health, contributing to detoxification.

7. Garlic:
   - Garlic contains sulfur compounds that support the production of glutathione, an antioxidant involved in detoxification.

8. Beets:

- o Beets contain betalains, which may support liver function and help eliminate toxins.
9. Green Tea:
   - o Green tea is rich in antioxidants, including catechins, which may have detoxifying effects.
10. Artichokes:
    - o Artichokes contain compounds that may support liver health and bile production, aiding in digestion and detoxification.
11. Cilantro:
    - o Cilantro has been studied for its potential to help eliminate heavy metals from the body.
12. Parsley:
    - o Parsley contains antioxidants and may support kidney function, contributing to detoxification.
13. Dandelion Greens:
    - o Dandelion greens may support liver health and act as a diuretic, promoting the elimination of toxins through urine.
14. Avocado:

- o Avocado contains glutathione, an antioxidant involved in the detoxification process.
15. Chia Seeds:
    - o Chia seeds are a good source of fiber, which supports digestive health and regular bowel movements.
16. Flaxseeds:
    - o Flaxseeds contain fiber and omega-3 fatty acids, supporting digestive health and overall well-being.
17. Mushrooms:
    - o Certain mushrooms, such as shiitake and maitake, contain compounds that may support immune function and detoxification.
18. Cabbage:
    - o Cabbage and other cruciferous vegetables contain sulfur compounds that support liver detoxification.

Including a variety of these foods in your diet, along with maintaining a well-balanced and nutrient-rich eating pattern, can contribute to supporting the body's natural detoxification processes. It's important to emphasize overall lifestyle habits, including hydration, regular physical activity, and stress management, for comprehensive well-being.

CRUCIFEROUS VEGETABLES

Vegetables in the Brassicaceae family are referred to as cruciferous vegetables. They are named for their cross-shaped flowers and are known for their distinct flavors and numerous health benefits. Here are some common cruciferous vegetables:

1. Broccoli:
    - Rich in vitamins C and K, as well as fiber, broccoli contains compounds like sulforaphane that have been associated with potential anti-cancer properties.
2. Cauliflower:
    - A versatile vegetable, cauliflower is low in calories and high in fiber.

It also contains sulforaphane and other beneficial compounds.

3. Cabbage:
    o Available in various varieties, including green, red, and Savoy cabbage, it is a good source of vitamins C and K, and it contains compounds that may have anti-inflammatory effects.
4. Brussels Sprouts:
    o These small, green vegetables are rich in vitamins A and C. They also provide fiber and contain glucosinolates, which can be converted into compounds with potential anti-cancer effects.
5. Kale:
    o A nutrient-dense leafy green, kale is high in vitamins A, C, and K, as well as minerals like calcium and potassium. It also has anti-inflammatory and antioxidant properties.
6. Arugula:
    o Arugula is a peppery, leafy green that is a good source of vitamins A, C, and K. It is also low in calories.

7. Bok Choy:
     - A common vegetable in Asian cuisine, bok choy is rich in vitamins A and C, as well as calcium and potassium.
8. Radishes:
     - Radishes are a crunchy root vegetable that adds a peppery flavor to salads. They are low in calories and provide small amounts of vitamins and minerals.
9. Turnips:
     - Turnips are root vegetables that can be cooked or eaten raw. They also have fiber and vitamins K and C.
10. Collard Greens:
     - Collard greens are leafy greens rich in vitamins A, C, and K. They also provide folate and manganese.

Cruciferous vegetables are known for their potential health benefits, including anti-inflammatory and antioxidant properties. In addition, they are linked to a lower risk of developing some types of cancer. Including a variety of these vegetables in your diet can contribute to overall health and well-being. Keep in mind that individual responses to foods can vary, and it's always a good idea to consume a diverse range of vegetables as part of a balanced diet.

HYDRATION

Staying hydrated is crucial for sustaining good health and a number of body processes. Here are key aspects of hydration and why it's crucial:

1. Fluid Balance:
   - Water helps maintain the balance of bodily fluids, which are essential for digestion, absorption, circulation, creation of saliva, nutrient transportation, and maintenance of body temperature.
2. Cellular Function:

- Adequate hydration is crucial for proper cellular function. Cells need water to carry out metabolic processes and transport nutrients and waste products.

3. Temperature Regulation:
   - One of the body's cooling techniques is sweating. Proper hydration helps regulate body temperature during physical activity or exposure to high temperatures.

4. Joint Lubrication:
   - Water acts as a lubricant for joints, helping reduce friction and discomfort during movement.

5. Nutrient Transport:
   - Water is a carrier for essential nutrients, transporting them throughout the body and facilitating their absorption.

6. Kidney Function:
   - When it comes to removing waste from the blood to create urine, the kidneys are essential. Adequate water intake supports optimal kidney function.

7. Cognitive Function:

- Cognitive function, including focus, alertness, and short-term memory, can be negatively impacted by dehydration.
8. Energy Levels:
    - Maintaining proper hydration levels helps sustain energy levels and can prevent feelings of fatigue.
9. Digestive Health:
    - Water is essential for digestion, helping break down food and move it through the digestive tract. Constipation may result from not drinking enough water.
10. Skin Health:
    - Hydration contributes to skin elasticity and a healthy complexion. Dehydration may lead to dry skin and an increased risk of skin issues.
11. Weight Management:
    - Drinking water before meals may contribute to a feeling of fullness, potentially supporting weight management by reducing calorie intake.
12. Exercise Performance:

- o Proper hydration is crucial for optimal athletic performance. Dehydration can lead to muscle cramps, fatigue, and impaired endurance.
13. Immune Function:
    - o Water plays a role in the production and circulation of lymph, which is involved in the immune system's defense against infections.
14. Detoxification:
    - o Adequate hydration supports the body's natural detoxification processes by aiding in the elimination of waste products.

It's generally recommended to drink about 8 glasses (64 ounces) of water per day, but individual water needs can vary based on factors such as age, weight, activity level, and climate. Thirst is a reliable indicator of your body's need for water, and it's essential to listen to your body's cues for proper hydration. Additionally, factors such as illness, pregnancy, and breastfeeding can influence hydration needs.

LIFESTYLE FACTORS

Lifestyle factors encompass a broad range of behaviors and choices that significantly impact overall health and well-being. Here are key lifestyle factors that contribute to a healthy and fulfilling life:

1. Nutritious Diet:
    - Eating a well-balanced diet rich in fruits, vegetables, whole grains, lean proteins, and healthy fats provides essential nutrients for optimal health.
2. Regular Physical Activity:
    - Engaging in regular exercise contributes to cardiovascular health, weight management, muscle strength, and overall well-being.
3. Adequate Sleep:
    - Good sleep is essential for both mental and physical well-being. It supports cognitive function, mood

regulation, and the body's natural healing processes.

4. Stress Management:
   - Employing stress-reducing techniques, such as meditation, deep breathing, yoga, or mindfulness, can promote mental and emotional well-being.

5. Hydration:
   - Maintaining proper hydration supports bodily functions, including digestion, circulation, and temperature regulation.

6. Avoiding Harmful Substances:
   - Limiting or avoiding tobacco, excessive alcohol, and recreational drugs reduces the risk of various health issues.

7. Maintaining a Healthy Weight:
   - Achieving and maintaining a healthy weight through a balanced diet and regular exercise contributes to overall health and reduces the risk of chronic diseases.

8. Social Connections:
   - Cultivating positive social relationships and maintaining a

supportive social network is vital for mental and emotional well-being.

9. Continual Learning:
   - Lifelong learning and intellectual stimulation contribute to cognitive health and personal growth.
10. Preventive Healthcare:
    - Regular health check-ups, screenings, and vaccinations are essential for preventive healthcare and early detection of potential issues.
11. Limiting Sedentary Behavior:
    - Minimizing prolonged periods of sitting and incorporating regular breaks for movement supports overall health.
12. Sun Protection:
    - Practicing sun safety, such as using sunscreen and protective clothing, helps prevent skin damage and reduces the risk of skin cancer.
13. Cultivating Hobbies:
    - Engaging in activities you enjoy, whether it's a hobby, sport, or

creative pursuit, contributes to a
fulfilling and balanced life.

14. Financial Well-Being:
    o Managing finances responsibly
      and planning for the future
      contributes to reduced stress and
      enhanced overall well-being.

15. Mindful Technology Use:
    o Balancing technology use and
      maintaining boundaries can
      support mental health and
      prevent digital burnout.

16. Environmental Awareness:
    o Being conscious of environmental
      impact and making sustainable
      choices contributes to personal
      and global well-being.

17. Cultural and Spiritual Engagement:
    o Exploring cultural interests and
      engaging in spiritual practices
      can provide a sense of purpose
      and fulfillment.

Adopting a holistic approach that considers
these lifestyle factors is key to promoting long-
term health and happiness. It's important to
note that individual needs and preferences

vary, so finding a balance that works for you is essential.

REGULAR PHYSICAL ACTIVITY

Regular physical activity is a cornerstone of a healthy lifestyle, offering a multitude of benefits for both physical and mental well-being. Here are key advantages of incorporating regular physical activity into your routine:

1. Cardiovascular Health:
   - Exercise lowers the risk of cardiovascular diseases like heart attacks and strokes by strengthening the heart and enhancing circulation.
2. Weight Management:
   - Regular physical activity, combined with a balanced diet, helps control weight and prevent obesity.
3. Muscle Strength and Endurance:
   - Engaging in resistance training and aerobic exercises improves

muscle strength, endurance, and overall physical performance.

4. Bone Health:
   o Weight-bearing exercises, like walking, running, and weightlifting, help maintain bone density and reduce the risk of osteoporosis.
5. Improved Mental Health:
   o Physical activity is linked to reduced symptoms of anxiety and depression. It releases endorphins, promoting feelings of happiness and relaxation.
6. Enhanced Flexibility and Balance:
   o Incorporating activities like stretching, yoga, and balance exercises enhances flexibility and reduces the risk of falls, especially in older adults.
7. Better Sleep:
   o Regular physical activity contributes to better sleep quality and can help alleviate insomnia.
8. Stress Reduction:
   o Exercise helps manage stress by reducing levels of stress

hormones and promoting
relaxation.

9. Improved Cognitive Function:
    - Physical activity is associated
      with better cognitive function,
      including improved memory and
      attention span.
10. Increased Energy Levels:
    - Frequent exercise increases
      vitality and decreases weariness.
11. Enhanced Immune Function:
    - Moderate physical activity may
      strengthen the immune system,
      reducing the risk of illness.
12. Social Interaction:
    - Group activities, sports, or
      exercise classes provide
      opportunities for social
      interaction, contributing to
      emotional well-being.
13. Prevention of Chronic Diseases:
    - Regular physical activity can help
      prevent or manage various
      chronic conditions, including type
      2 diabetes, hypertension, and
      certain cancers.
14. Longevity:

- Studies suggest that regular exercise is associated with a longer life expectancy.

15. Mood Regulation:
    - Physical activity can positively impact mood by promoting the release of neurotransmitters like serotonin and dopamine.

16. Better Posture:
    - Engaging in exercises that target core strength and flexibility contributes to improved posture.

17. Enhanced Self-Esteem:
    - Achieving fitness goals and engaging in regular physical activity can boost self-confidence and self-esteem.

It's important to choose activities you enjoy to make regular physical activity a sustainable part of your lifestyle. The American Heart Association recommends at least 150 minutes of moderate-intensity exercise or 75 minutes of vigorous-intensity exercise per week, along with muscle-strengthening activities at least two days a week.

STRESS MANAGEMENT

Effective stress management is crucial for maintaining overall well-being and mitigating the negative effects of stress on physical and mental health. The following techniques can be used to control and lessen stress:

1. Deep Breathing:
    - To trigger the relaxation response in your body, engage in deep breathing exercises. Breathe in deeply through your nose, hold it for a short while, and then slowly release the air through your mouth.
2. Mindfulness Meditation:
    - Engage in mindfulness meditation to focus your attention on the present moment, promoting a sense of calm and reducing stress.
3. Physical Activity:
    - Regular exercise helps release endorphins, the body's natural stress relievers. Exercises like

yoga, jogging, and walking can
be advantageous.

4. Progressive Muscle Relaxation (PMR):
    - PMR involves tensing and then gradually releasing each muscle group to promote relaxation throughout the body.
5. Healthy Lifestyle Choices:
    - Maintain a balanced diet, prioritize adequate sleep, and limit the consumption of stimulants like caffeine and alcohol to support overall well-being.
6. Time Management:
    - Organize your schedule, set realistic goals, and prioritize tasks to reduce feelings of overwhelm and stress.
7. Social Support:
    - To express emotions and get emotional support, get in touch with friends, family, or support groups. Having social ties is crucial for stress resilience.
8. Nature and Outdoor Activities:
    - Participate in outdoor activities or spend time in nature. The mind

can be calmed by being in an environment with natural surroundings and fresh air.

9. Art and Creative Expression:
    - Engage in creative activities like drawing, painting, writing, or playing music as a way to express emotions and relieve stress.

10. Limiting Stimuli:
    - Reduce exposure to stressors such as excessive noise, screen time, or information overload. Take breaks from technology when needed.

11. Laughter and Humor:
    - Laughter triggers the release of endorphins and can provide a natural and immediate stress relief.

12. Mindful Eating:
    - Pay attention to what and how you eat. Eating mindfully can promote relaxation and help maintain a healthy relationship with food.

13. Cognitive Behavioral Techniques:

- Practice cognitive restructuring by challenging negative thought patterns and replacing them with more positive and realistic perspectives.

14. Journaling:
    - Keep a journal where you can record your feelings and thoughts. Reflecting on your experiences can help gain insight and alleviate stress.

15. Self-Compassion:
    - Be kind to yourself. Treating yourself with the same consideration and understanding that you would extend to a friend is a great way to practice self-compassion.

16. Seeking Professional Support:
    - If stress becomes overwhelming, consider seeking support from a mental health professional, such as a counselor or therapist.

Keep in mind that everyone reacts to stress in different ways. It's important to explore and identify strategies that work best for you.

Consistency in incorporating stress management techniques into your routine can contribute to long-term resilience and well-being.

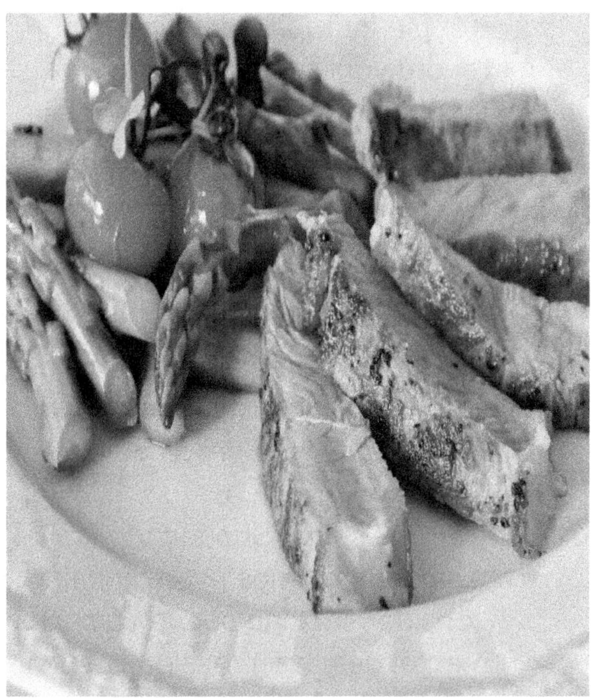

CHAPTER 4

WEIGHT MANAGEMENT FOR WOMEN OVER 40

Weight management for women over 40 involves a combination of healthy eating, regular physical activity, and lifestyle adjustments. Here are some tips to support weight management in this age group:

1. Balanced Nutrition:
    - Focus on a well-balanced diet that includes a variety of nutrient-dense foods such as fruits, vegetables, whole grains, lean proteins, and healthy fats. To manage your intake of calories, think about portion control.
2. Protein Intake:
    - Ensure an adequate intake of protein, which is crucial for maintaining muscle mass, especially as metabolism tends to slow down with age. Include sources like lean meats, fish,

dairy, eggs, legumes, and plant-based proteins.

3. Hydration:
    - Stay well-hydrated by drinking water throughout the day. Thirst can occasionally be mistaken for hunger.

4. Fiber-Rich Foods:
    - Include fiber in your diet through whole grains, fruits, vegetables, and legumes. Fiber helps with digestion, promotes a feeling of fullness, and supports weight management.

5. Limit Processed Foods and Added Sugars:
    - Minimize the intake of processed foods and foods high in added sugars, as they can contribute to excess calorie consumption.

6. Regular Physical Activity:
    - Engage in a combination of aerobic exercises (e.g., walking, jogging, swimming) and strength training to boost metabolism, maintain muscle mass, and promote overall fitness.

7. Strength Training:

- Incorporate exercises for strength training to develop and preserve muscle. This is especially important for women over 40, as muscle mass tends to decrease with age.

8. Mindful Eating:
   - Pay attention to hunger and fullness cues. Eating mindfully, without distractions, can help prevent overeating.

9. Adequate Sleep:
   - Prioritize getting enough quality sleep. Hormones linked to appetite and hunger can be impacted by sleep deprivation.

10. Stress Management:
    - Use stress-reduction methods like yoga, deep breathing, and meditation. Chronic stress can impact weight and overall health.

11. Regular Health Check-ups:
    - Consult with healthcare professionals regularly to monitor health and address any underlying conditions that may affect weight management.

12. Hormone Health:

- Hormonal changes during perimenopause and menopause can affect weight distribution. Discuss hormone-related concerns with a healthcare provider.

13. Consistency is Key:
    - Establish sustainable habits and be consistent in your approach to nutrition and exercise. Gradual, long-term changes are more effective than quick fixes.

14. Social Support:
    - Share your health and fitness goals with friends or family for support. The journey can be more successful and enjoyable if you have a support system.

15. Be Patient and Realistic:
    - Weight management is a gradual process. Set attainable objectives and acknowledge minor accomplishments along the way. Pay attention to your general health and well-being rather than just the scale's number.

It's important to note that individual responses to diet and exercise can vary, and it's advisable to consult with healthcare professionals or registered dietitians for personalized guidance based on individual health needs and goals.

METABOLISM SUPPORT

Supporting metabolism is crucial for maintaining energy levels and managing weight. Here are lifestyle and dietary strategies that may help boost metabolism:

1. Regular Physical Activity:
   - Engage in both aerobic exercises (e.g., walking, jogging, cycling) and strength training to increase muscle mass. Muscle tissue burns more calories at rest, contributing to a higher metabolism.
2. High-Intensity Interval Training (HIIT):
   - Incorporate short bursts of intense exercise followed by rest periods. HIIT has been shown to

boost metabolism and improve
cardiovascular health.
3. Strength Training:
    o Include resistance or strength
      training exercises at least two to
      three times per week. Building
      and maintaining muscle mass
      can enhance metabolism.
4. Adequate Protein Intake:
    o When it comes to digestion,
      protein needs more energy than
      fats and carbohydrates. Including
      lean protein sources in meals can
      temporarily increase calorie
      expenditure.
5. Stay Hydrated:
    o Drinking water is essential for
      metabolic processes. Your
      metabolism can be slowed down
      by even slight dehydration.
6. Green Tea:
    o Green tea has ingredients like
      catechins that could speed up
      metabolism. Consider
      incorporating it into your routine
      for added health benefits.
7. Adequate Sleep:

- Lack of sleep can negatively impact metabolism and hormonal regulation. Aim for 7-9 hours of quality sleep per night.

8. Manage Stress:
   - Chronic stress can elevate cortisol levels, affecting metabolism. Use stress-reduction strategies like yoga, deep breathing, and meditation.

9. Spicy Foods:
   - Capsaicin, found in chili peppers, may have a temporary thermogenic effect, potentially increasing calorie expenditure.

10. Omega-3 Fatty Acids:
    - Foods rich in omega-3 fatty acids, such as fatty fish, flaxseeds, and walnuts, may support metabolic health.

11. Fiber-Rich Foods:
    - High-fiber foods like fruits, vegetables, and whole grains can contribute to a feeling of fullness and may have a modest effect on metabolism.

12. Regular Meals:

- o Eat regular, balanced meals throughout the day. Skipping meals can lead to a slowdown in metabolism.
13. Intermittent Fasting:
    - o Some studies suggest that intermittent fasting may influence metabolism and improve insulin sensitivity.
14. Cold Exposure:
    - o Exposure to cold temperatures may stimulate brown fat, a type of fat that burns calories to generate heat. Cold showers or spending time in a cool environment might have a modest impact.
15. Coffee:
    - o Caffeine, found in coffee, can temporarily boost metabolic rate. However, it's essential to consume it in moderation and be mindful of individual tolerance.

It's important to note that individual responses to these strategies can vary, and there's no one-size-fits-all approach. Adopting a combination of these lifestyle and dietary habits, tailored to individual needs and preferences, can contribute to overall metabolic health.

HORMONAL BALANCE THROUGH DIET

Hormone balance must be maintained for general health and wellbeing. While diet alone may not completely regulate hormones, certain dietary practices can support hormonal balance. Here are some tips to promote hormonal health through diet:

1. Balanced Nutrition:
    - Eat a range of whole foods, such as fruits, vegetables, whole grains, lean meats, and healthy fats, as part of a diet that is well-balanced. Nutrient-dense foods provide essential vitamins and minerals that support overall health, including hormonal function.
2. Adequate Protein:
    - Include sufficient protein in your diet, as it is essential for the production and regulation of

hormones. Tofu, fish, beans, lentils, and poultry are examples of foods high in lean protein.

3. Healthy Fats:
   - Include heart-healthy fats like those in olive oil, avocados, nuts, and seeds. These fats are precursors to hormones and contribute to hormonal balance.
4. Omega-3 Fatty Acids:
   - Add foods high in omega-3 fatty acids, like walnuts, flaxseeds, chia seeds, and fatty fish (salmon, mackerel). Omega-3s are crucial for various hormonal functions.
5. Complex Carbohydrates:
   - Choose complex carbohydrates like whole grains, brown rice, quinoa, and sweet potatoes. These provide sustained energy and support stable blood sugar levels, which is important for hormonal balance.
6. Fiber-Rich Foods:
   - High-fiber foods, including fruits, vegetables, and legumes, support digestive health and may

help regulate insulin levels, impacting hormonal balance.

7. Colorful Vegetables:
   - Eat a variety of colorful vegetables to benefit from a range of antioxidants and phytonutrients. These compounds support overall health, including hormonal function.

8. Probiotic-Rich Foods:
   - Incorporate foods high in probiotics, such as kimchi, kefir, yogurt, and sauerkraut. Hormonal balance and gut microbiome health are related.

9. Limit Processed Foods:
   - Reduce the intake of processed foods, which may contain added sugars, unhealthy fats, and artificial additives that can disrupt hormonal balance.

10. Moderate Caffeine and Alcohol:
    - Limit caffeine and alcohol intake, as excessive amounts can affect hormone levels. Opt for moderation and be mindful of individual tolerance.

11. Hydration:
    o Stay well-hydrated by drinking water throughout the day. Proper hydration is essential for hormonal and overall health.
12. Manage Sugar Intake:
    o Be mindful of added sugars in your diet. High sugar consumption can lead to insulin resistance, impacting hormonal balance.
13. Limit Trans Fats:
    o Avoid or minimize trans fats found in some processed and fried foods, as they can negatively impact hormone regulation.
14. Sufficient Caloric Intake:
    o Ensure you're consuming enough calories to support your energy needs. A severe calorie restriction may throw off the balance of hormones.
15. Adaptogenic Herbs:
    o Some herbs, such as ashwagandha and rhodiola, are considered adaptogens that may

help the body adapt to stress and support hormonal balance.

PORTION CONTROL AND MINDFUL EATING

Portion control and mindful eating are important practices that can contribute to a healthy relationship with food and support overall well-being. Here's a breakdown of both concepts:

Portion Control:

1. Understand Serving Sizes:
   - Learn the appropriate serving sizes for each of the food groups. This helps you gauge appropriate portions.
2. Use Smaller Plates and Bowls:
   - Opt for smaller dishes to visually trick your mind into feeling satisfied with smaller portions.
3. Divide Your Plate:
   - Mentally divide your plate into sections for proteins, carbohydrates, and vegetables.

This can guide you to create a balanced meal.

4. Avoid Second Helpings Immediately:
    - Allow some time to pass before considering a second serving. This helps your body signal whether it's truly hungry for more.

5. Be Mindful of Liquid Calories:
    - Be aware of the calories in beverages. Sugary drinks and excessive alcohol intake can contribute significantly to overall calorie intake.

6. Read Food Labels:
    - Check nutrition labels for information on serving sizes and calories per serving. This will enable you to make wise decisions.

7. Pre-Portion Snacks:
    - Instead of eating directly from the package, pre-portion snacks into smaller containers to avoid overeating.

8. Listen to Hunger Cues:
    - Take note of your body's hunger and fullness cues. Don't overeat; just until you're satisfied.

Mindful Eating:

1. Eat Without Distractions:
   - Avoid eating in front of the TV or computer. Focus on the sensory experience of eating, including flavors, textures, and smells.
2. Chew Thoroughly:
   - Chew your food slowly and thoroughly. This not only aids digestion but also allows your brain to register signals of fullness.
3. Savor Each Bite:
   - Give each bite due appreciation and savoring. This can enhance the enjoyment of your meal and help you recognize when you're satisfied.
4. Check-in with Hunger Levels:
   - Before eating, assess your hunger level. Are you eating out of habit, boredom, or true hunger?
5. Use All Your Senses:
   - Engage all your senses while eating. Take note of your food's flavors, textures, and colors. This

brings awareness to the eating experience.

6. Pause Between Bites:
   - Put your utensils down between bites. This slows down your eating pace and allows your body to signal when it's satisfied.
7. Recognize Emotional Eating:
   - Be mindful of emotional triggers for eating. If you're eating for reasons other than hunger, consider alternative ways to address those emotions.
8. Express Gratitude:
   - Give yourself a moment to be thankful for your dinner. This positive mindset can contribute to a more mindful eating experience.
9. Be Non-Judgmental:
   - Avoid labeling foods as "good" or "bad." Allow yourself to enjoy a variety of foods without guilt or judgment.

Combining portion control with mindful eating can foster a healthy relationship with food, promote better digestion, and contribute to weight management. It's important to be patient and make these practices a gradual part of your routine for long-term success.

INCORPORATING REGULAR EXERCISE

Incorporating regular exercise into your routine is a key component of a healthy lifestyle, offering numerous physical and mental health benefits. Here are some tips to help you make exercise a consistent part of your daily life:

1. Set Realistic Goals:
    - Establish achievable and realistic fitness goals. Whether it's walking for 30 minutes a day or completing a weekly workout routine, setting specific goals provides direction.
2. Find Activities You Enjoy:
    - Choose exercises or activities that you find enjoyable. Whether it's dancing, hiking, swimming, or playing a sport, selecting

activities you like increases the likelihood of sticking with them.

3. Start Gradually:
    - If you're new to exercise or returning after a break, start with manageable durations and intensities. Increase the duration and intensity gradually as your fitness level rises.
4. Make it a Routine:
    - Schedule specific times for your workouts, treating them as appointments. Consistency is key in building a habit.
5. Mix Up Your Workouts:
    - Use a range of exercises to keep things interesting. This works various muscle groups and helps avoid boredom.
6. Include Strength Training:
    - Integrate strength training exercises at least two to three times a week. Building and maintaining muscle mass is crucial for overall health.
7. Involve Friends or Family:
    - Exercise with friends or family members. Not only does this

make it more enjoyable, but it also provides mutual motivation and accountability.

8. Utilize Technology:
   - Use fitness apps, wearables, or online workout programs to track your progress and stay motivated. Many apps offer guided workouts and allow you to set fitness goals.
9. Prioritize Consistency Over Intensity:
   - Consistent, moderate-intensity exercise can have significant health benefits. It's more important to establish a routine that you can maintain over time rather than pushing yourself too hard initially.
10. Listen to Your Body:
    - Observe how your body reacts to physical activity. Allow time for rest and recovery when needed, and don't hesitate to modify your routine based on how you feel.
11. Set Non-Fitness Goals:
    - Consider setting non-fitness-related goals that exercise can help you achieve. Whether it's

stress reduction, improved sleep,
or increased energy levels,
connecting exercise to broader
goals can enhance motivation.

12. Celebrate Achievements:
    - No matter how tiny, recognize
      and celebrate your fitness
      accomplishments.
      Acknowledging your development
      can increase self-assurance and
      motivation.

13. Join Classes or Groups:
    - Participate in fitness classes or
      join exercise groups. The social
      aspect can make workouts more
      enjoyable and provide a sense of
      community.

14. Be Flexible:
    - Recognize that life can be
      unpredictable. If you miss a
      workout or face a scheduling
      challenge, be flexible and find
      alternative ways to stay active.

15. Consult a Professional:
    - If you have specific health
      concerns or fitness goals,
      consider consulting with a fitness

professional or personal trainer to
create a tailored exercise plan.

Remember that any amount of physical activity
is better than none, and finding ways to move
that you enjoy will contribute to your overall
well-being.

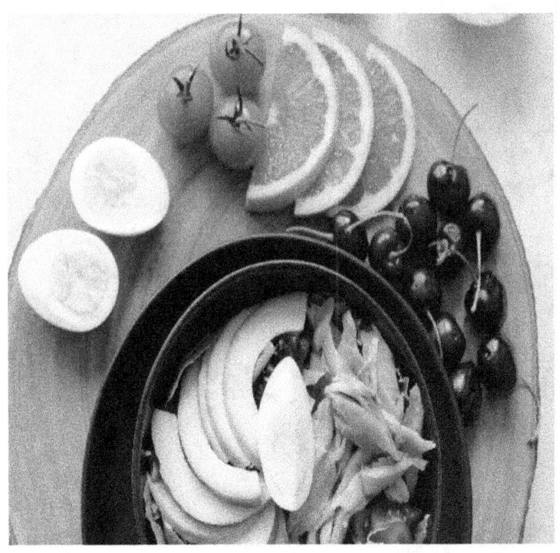

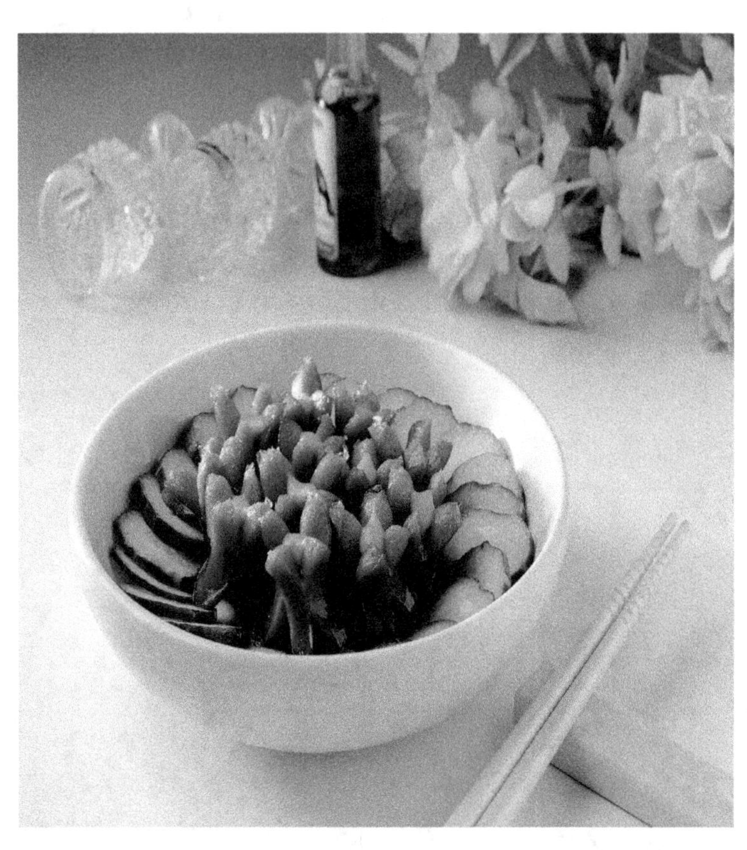

CHAPTER 5

SAMPLE 14-DAYS MEAL PLAN

Here's a sample 14-day meal plan focused on balanced nutrition, supporting healthy aging, and incorporating immune-boosting components. This plan includes a variety of nutrient-dense foods, lean proteins, whole grains, fruits, and vegetables. Remember to adapt portion sizes based on your individual needs and preferences.

Day 1:

- Breakfast:
    - Greek yogurt parfait with mixed berries and a sprinkle of chia seeds.
- Lunch:
    - Grilled chicken salad with mixed greens, cherry tomatoes, cucumber, and a vinaigrette dressing.
- Dinner:
    - Baked salmon with quinoa and roasted vegetables (e.g.,

broccoli, carrots, and bell peppers).

Day 2:

- Breakfast:
    - Oatmeal topped with sliced banana, almonds, and a drizzle of honey.
- Lunch:
    - Quinoa and black bean bowl with avocado, salsa, and a side of mixed greens.
- Dinner:
    - Stir-fried tofu with brown rice and a variety of colorful vegetables.

Day 3:

- Breakfast:
    - Whole grain toast with avocado, poached eggs, and a side of grapefruit.
- Lunch:
    - Lentil soup with a side of whole grain crackers and a green salad.

- Dinner:
  - Grilled shrimp with sweet potato wedges and steamed asparagus.

Day 4:

- Breakfast:
  - Smoothie with spinach, banana, berries, Greek yogurt, and a scoop of protein powder.
- Lunch:
  - Quinoa salad with cherry tomatoes, feta cheese, olives, and a lemon vinaigrette.
- Dinner:
  - Baked chicken breast with wild rice and sautéed green beans.

Day 5:

- Breakfast:
  - Whole grain English muffin with smoked salmon, cream cheese, and sliced cucumber.
- Lunch:

- Chickpea and vegetable stir-fry with brown rice.
  - Dinner:
    - Turkey meatballs with whole wheat pasta and tomato sauce.

Day 6:

- Breakfast:
  - Cottage cheese with pineapple chunks and a sprinkle of sunflower seeds.
- Lunch:
  - Quinoa-stuffed bell peppers with a side of mixed greens.
- Dinner:
  - Grilled cod with quinoa pilaf and roasted Brussels sprouts.

Day 7:

- Breakfast:
  - Whole grain pancakes with fresh berries and a dollop of Greek yogurt.
- Lunch:

- ○ Lentil and vegetable curry with brown rice.
- Dinner:
  - ○ Beef and vegetable kebabs with sweet potato fries.

Day 8-14:

Repeat the above meal ideas, mixing and matching to create a variety of meals throughout the week. Don't forget to stay hydrated with water, herbal teas, and incorporate snacks like nuts, fruits, or veggies between meals as needed.

Adjust the plan based on your dietary preferences, any food allergies or intolerances, and individual nutritional requirements.

BREAKFAST OPTIONS

Here are various breakfast options that you can incorporate into your meal plan for a balanced and nutritious start to the day:

1. Greek Yogurt Parfait:
    o Layer Greek yogurt with fresh berries, granola, and a drizzle of honey.
2. Oatmeal with Toppings:
    o Cooked oats topped with sliced bananas, chopped nuts, and a sprinkle of cinnamon.
3. Avocado Toast with Poached Eggs:
    o Whole grain toast topped with mashed avocado and poached eggs. Season with salt and pepper.
4. Smoothie Bowl:
    o Blend your favorite fruits, greens, and a scoop of protein powder. Top with granola, chia seeds, and sliced almonds.
5. Whole Grain Pancakes:
    o Enjoy whole grain pancakes topped with fresh berries and a dollop of Greek yogurt.
6. Egg and Veggie Scramble:
    o Scrambled eggs with sautéed vegetables like spinach, tomatoes, and bell peppers.
7. Chia Seed Pudding:

o   Mix chia seeds with almond milk and let it sit overnight. Top with sliced strawberries and a drizzle of maple syrup.

8. Breakfast Burrito:
    o   Whole grain tortilla filled with scrambled eggs, black beans, salsa, and avocado.
9. Cottage Cheese Bowl:
    o   Cottage cheese with sliced pineapple, a handful of sunflower seeds, and a sprinkle of cinnamon.
10. Whole Grain Bagel with Smoked Salmon:
    o   Whole grain bagel topped with cream cheese, smoked salmon, and sliced cucumber.
11. Quinoa Breakfast Bowl:
    o   Quinoa cooked in milk with vanilla extract, topped with mixed berries and a dollop of yogurt.
12. Peanut Butter Banana Toast:
    o   Whole grain toast with peanut butter and sliced bananas.
13. Breakfast Wrap:

- Whole grain wrap filled with scrambled eggs, spinach, feta cheese, and cherry tomatoes.
14. Fruit Salad with Cottage Cheese:
    - Fresh fruit salad with a side of cottage cheese for added protein.
15. Egg Muffins:
    - Whisk eggs and pour into muffin cups with diced vegetables. Bake for a quick and portable breakfast.

Remember to tailor these options based on your dietary preferences, nutritional needs, and any food allergies or intolerances you may have. Balancing carbohydrates, proteins, and healthy fats in your breakfast can help provide sustained energy throughout the morning.

LUNCH IDEAS

Here are various lunch ideas that you can incorporate into your meal plan for a nutritious and satisfying midday meal:

1. Grilled Chicken Salad:

- Mixed greens with grilled chicken breast, cherry tomatoes, cucumber, and a light vinaigrette dressing.
2. Quinoa and Black Bean Bowl:
   - Quinoa mixed with black beans, corn, avocado, salsa, and a squeeze of lime.
3. Lentil Soup with Whole Grain Crackers:
   - Hearty lentil soup served with a side of whole grain crackers.
4. Turkey and Veggie Wrap:
   - Whole grain wrap with sliced turkey, hummus, shredded carrots, and spinach.
5. Chickpea and Vegetable Stir-Fry:
   - Stir-fried chickpeas with a colorful mix of vegetables served over brown rice.
6. Caprese Salad Sandwich:
   - Whole grain bread with fresh mozzarella, tomato slices, basil, and a drizzle of balsamic glaze.
7. Quinoa Salad with Feta:
   - Quinoa salad with feta cheese, cherry tomatoes, olives, and a lemon vinaigrette.
8. Tuna Salad Lettuce Wraps:

- Tuna salad made with light mayo, celery, and onions, wrapped in lettuce leaves.

9. Vegetarian Buddha Bowl:
   - Brown rice or quinoa with roasted sweet potatoes, kale, chickpeas, and tahini dressing.
10. Mediterranean Couscous Salad:
    - Couscous salad with cucumbers, cherry tomatoes, Kalamata olives, and feta cheese.
11. Chicken and Vegetable Skewers:
    - Grilled chicken skewers with bell peppers, zucchini, and cherry tomatoes.
12. Salmon and Avocado Wrap:
    - Whole grain wrap with smoked salmon, avocado, cream cheese, and arugula.
13. Veggie-Packed Minestrone Soup:
    - Minestrone soup loaded with a variety of vegetables and whole grain pasta.
14. Tofu Stir-Fry with Broccoli:
    - Stir-fried tofu with broccoli, snow peas, and carrots served over brown rice.
15. Egg Salad Lettuce Wraps:

    ○ Egg salad made with Greek yogurt, mustard, and chives, wrapped in lettuce leaves.

16. Shrimp and Quinoa Bowl:
    ○ Quinoa bowl with sautéed shrimp, black beans, corn, and avocado.
17. Chopped Chicken Caesar Salad:
    ○ Chopped romaine lettuce with grilled chicken, cherry tomatoes, croutons, and Caesar dressing.
18. Veggie Burger with Sweet Potato Fries:
    ○ Veggie burger on a whole grain bun with lettuce, tomato, and a side of baked sweet potato fries.
19. Pita Bread with Hummus and Veggies:
    ○ Whole wheat pita filled with hummus, cucumber, cherry tomatoes, and red onion.
20. Roasted Vegetable Wrap:
    ○ Roasted vegetables (bell peppers, zucchini, and eggplant) in a whole grain wrap with a drizzle of balsamic glaze.

Feel free to mix and match these ideas, and adapt them based on your taste preferences and dietary needs. Remember to consider portion sizes and include a variety of colorful vegetables for a well-balanced and satisfying lunch.

DINNER RECIPES

Here are various dinner recipes that you can incorporate into your meal plan for delicious and nutritious evening meals:

1. Baked Lemon Garlic Salmon:
    - Baked salmon fillets with a marinade of lemon, garlic, and herbs. Serve with quinoa and steamed asparagus.
2. Vegetarian Stir-Fried Noodles:
    - Stir-fried noodles with tofu, broccoli, bell peppers, and snow peas in a flavorful soy-ginger sauce.
3. Grilled Chicken with Mediterranean Quinoa:
    - Grilled chicken breasts seasoned with Mediterranean herbs, served over quinoa with cherry

tomatoes, olives, and feta
cheese.
4. Spaghetti Bolognese:
    o Whole wheat spaghetti with a rich
       tomato and lentil-based
       Bolognese sauce. Top with
       grated Parmesan.
5. Vegetable and Chickpea Curry:
    o A hearty curry with a mix of
       vegetables and chickpeas in a
       coconut milk and curry spice
       sauce. Serve over brown rice.
6. Teriyaki Glazed Tofu Stir-Fry:
    o Stir-fried tofu, broccoli, carrots,
       and snap peas in a homemade
       teriyaki glaze. Serve over brown
       rice or quinoa.
7. Grilled Vegetable and Quinoa Stuffed
   Peppers:
    o Bell peppers stuffed with a
       mixture of quinoa, black beans,
       corn, and grilled vegetables,
       baked to perfection.
8. Mushroom and Spinach Risotto:
    o Creamy risotto made with Arborio
       rice, mushrooms, spinach, and a
       touch of Parmesan cheese.
9. Healthy Chicken Caesar Salad:

- Grilled chicken slices on a bed of romaine lettuce with cherry tomatoes, whole grain croutons, and a light Caesar dressing.

10. Chickpea and Sweet Potato Curry:
    - A comforting curry with chickpeas, sweet potatoes, and spinach in a coconut milk and curry sauce. Serve over brown rice.

11. Baked Cod with Tomato Salsa:
    - Baked cod fillets topped with a fresh tomato salsa. Serve with quinoa and steamed green beans.

12. Veggie-Packed Fajitas:
    - Colorful bell peppers, onions, and your choice of protein (chicken, beef, or tofu) seasoned with fajita spices. Serve in whole wheat tortillas.

13. Shrimp and Vegetable Skewers:
    - Skewers with shrimp, cherry tomatoes, zucchini, and red onion, grilled and served over couscous.

14. Lentil and Vegetable Stuffed Bell Peppers:

- Bell peppers stuffed with a mixture of lentils, quinoa, tomatoes, and spices. Baked until tender.

15. Mango Salsa Chicken:
    - Grilled chicken breasts topped with a refreshing mango salsa. Serve with brown rice or quinoa.

16. Spinach and Feta Stuffed Chicken Breast:
    - Chicken breasts stuffed with a mixture of spinach and feta cheese, baked to perfection.

17. Healthy Beef and Broccoli Stir-Fry:
    - Stir-fried lean beef strips with broccoli and carrots in a savory ginger-soy sauce. Serve over brown rice.

18. Eggplant Parmesan:
    - Baked slices of eggplant layered with marinara sauce and mozzarella cheese. Serve with a side of whole wheat pasta.

19. Turkey and Vegetable Chili:
    - Lean ground turkey chili with kidney beans, tomatoes, and a blend of spices. Top with Greek

yogurt and chopped green
onions.

20. Quinoa Stuffed Acorn Squash:
    ○ Roasted acorn squash halves
      filled with quinoa, black beans,
      corn, and diced tomatoes.

Feel free to customize these recipes based on your dietary preferences and portion sizes. Cooking at home allows you to control ingredients and make meals that suit your taste while providing essential nutrients.

SNACK SUGGESTIONS

Here are some healthy snack suggestions that you can enjoy between meals:

1. Greek Yogurt with Berries:
    ○ A serving of Greek yogurt with
      fresh berries (strawberries,
      blueberries, or raspberries).
2. Apple Slices with Almond Butter:
    ○ Apple slices paired with a
      tablespoon of almond butter for a

satisfying combination of crunch
and creaminess.
3. Hummus and Veggie Sticks:
    o   Carrot, cucumber, and bell
        pepper sticks with a side of
        hummus for a nutritious and
        flavorful snack.
4. Mixed Nuts and Dried Fruits:
    o   A small handful of mixed nuts
        (almonds, walnuts, or pistachios)
        with dried fruits like apricots or
        raisins.
5. Cheese and Whole Grain Crackers:
    o   A portion of your favorite cheese
        paired with whole grain crackers
        for a balanced and satisfying
        snack.
6. Hard-Boiled Eggs:
    o   Hard-boiled eggs are a protein-
        packed and portable snack.
7. Smoothie:
    o   Blend together your favorite
        fruits, vegetables, Greek yogurt,
        and a splash of almond milk for a
        refreshing smoothie.
8. Cherry Tomatoes with Mozzarella Balls:

- Cherry tomatoes paired with mini mozzarella balls for a quick and tasty bite.

9. Oatmeal Energy Bites:
   - Homemade energy bites made with oats, nut butter, honey, and add-ins like chia seeds or dark chocolate chips.

10. Edamame:
    - Steamed edamame sprinkled with a touch of sea salt for a protein-rich and satisfying snack.

11. Cottage Cheese with Pineapple:
    - Cottage cheese topped with fresh pineapple chunks for a sweet and savory treat.

12. Popcorn:
    - Air-popped popcorn seasoned with a sprinkle of nutritional yeast or your favorite herbs for a light and crunchy snack.

13. Avocado Rice Cakes:
    - Rice cakes topped with sliced avocado, a dash of salt, and a sprinkle of red pepper flakes.

14. Yogurt Parfait:

- Layer low-fat yogurt with granola and mixed berries for a delicious and textured parfait.

15. Trail Mix:
    - Make your own trail mix with a mix of nuts, seeds, and dried fruits. Add a touch of dark chocolate for sweetness.

16. Veggies and Guacamole:
    - Sliced veggies (like bell peppers or cucumber) served with homemade guacamole.

17. Whole Grain Toast with Nut Butter:
    - Whole grain toast spread with your favorite nut butter (peanut butter, almond butter, or cashew butter).

18. Berries with Cottage Cheese:
    - Cottage cheese topped with a medley of fresh berries for a protein-rich and antioxidant-packed snack.

19. Chia Seed Pudding:
    - Chia seed pudding made with almond milk and topped with sliced fruit or a drizzle of honey.

20. Rice Cake with Tuna Salad:

- Tuna salad (canned tuna, Greek yogurt, celery, and spices) on a rice cake for a satisfying and protein-rich option.

Remember to pay attention to portion sizes, and these snacks can be tailored based on your preferences and dietary needs. Enjoying a variety of nutrient-dense snacks throughout the day can help keep your energy levels steady and curb hunger between meals.

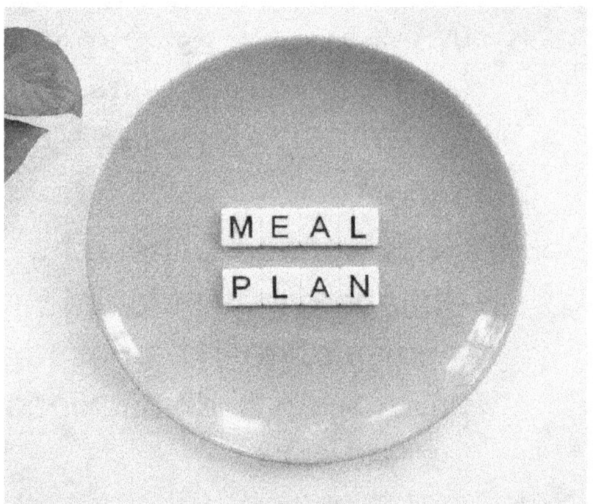

CHAPTER 6

ADDITIONAL TIPS FOR SUCCESS

Here are additional tips to enhance your success in adopting a healthy and balanced lifestyle:

1. Stay Hydrated:
   - Drink plenty of water throughout the day. Hydration is crucial for overall health and can help control hunger.
2. Practice Mindful Eating:
   - Pay attention to your eating habits. Eat mindfully, enjoy every bite, and pay attention to your body's signals of hunger and fullness.
3. Plan and Prepare:
   - Plan your meals and snacks in advance. You can choose healthier options and maintain control over the ingredients when you prepare meals at home.
4. Get Quality Sleep:

- Every night, try to get seven to nine hours of good sleep. Sleep is essential for overall well-being and can impact your food choices and energy levels.

5. Manage Stress:
   - Incorporate stress-reducing activities into your routine, such as meditation, deep breathing exercises, or activities you enjoy.

6. Set Realistic Goals:
   - Set achievable and realistic goals for yourself. Segment more complex objectives into more doable smaller ones.

7. Variety is Key:
   - To guarantee that your diet contains a wide range of nutrients, include a variety of foods. Explore new fruits, vegetables, and whole grains.

8. Listen to Your Body:
   - Take note of your feelings after eating various foods. Based on what suits your unique needs and preferences, modify your diet.

9. Celebrate Progress:

- Celebrate your successes, no matter how small. Acknowledge and reward yourself for sticking to healthy habits.

10. Stay Active Throughout the Day:
    - Incorporate movement into your daily routine. Take short walks, use stairs, or do quick home workouts to stay active.

11. Accountability:
    - Consider sharing your health goals with a friend or family member for mutual support and accountability.

12. Be Patient:
    - Building healthy habits takes time. Practice self-compassion and concentrate on implementing small, long-lasting adjustments.

13. Limit Processed Foods:
    - Reduce your intake of processed and refined foods. Opt for whole, nutrient-dense options whenever possible.

14. Read Food Labels:
    - Get acquainted with food labels so that you can choose the products you buy with

knowledge. Pay attention to serving sizes and nutritional content.

15. Social Support:
    - Surround yourself with a supportive community. Whether online or in-person, having people to share your journey with can be motivating.

16. Regular Check-Ins:
    - Evaluate your progress on a regular basis and revise your plan as necessary. This can assist you in staying on course and pinpointing areas that need work.

17. Be Flexible:
    - Life can be unpredictable. Be flexible and adapt to changes without feeling discouraged. When faced with obstacles, look for different ways to solve the problem.

18. Educate Yourself:
    - Stay informed about nutrition and health. Understanding the benefits of your choices can reinforce positive habits.

19. Reward Yourself Mindfully:
    ○ Instead of using food as a reward, consider non-food rewards like a relaxing bath, a book you've been wanting to read, or a favorite hobby.
20. Consult with Professionals:
    ○ If you have specific health concerns or goals, consider seeking guidance from a healthcare professional, nutritionist, or fitness trainer.

Remember, the journey to a healthier lifestyle is unique to each individual. Find what works best for you, and make changes gradually to ensure long-term success.

MEAL PREPPING

Meal prepping is a fantastic way to save time, make healthier food choices, and stay on track with your nutrition. Here are some pointers for effective meal planning:

1. Plan Your Meals:

- Outline your meals for the week, considering a balance of proteins, vegetables, whole grains, and healthy fats.

2. Choose a Prep Day:
   - Every week, set aside a particular day to prepare meals. This helps streamline the process and ensures you have meals ready to go.
3. Create a Menu:
   - Develop a menu for the week, including breakfast, lunch, dinner, and snacks. This makes your grocery shopping more efficient.
4. Keep it Balanced:
   - Ensure your meals include a variety of nutrients. Aim for a mix of lean proteins, colorful vegetables, whole grains, and healthy fats.
5. Invest in Quality Containers:
   - Invest in a variety of durable and reusable containers. This makes it easy to portion and store your meals.
6. Batch Cooking:

- Cook large batches of proteins (chicken, beans, quinoa) and grains to use in multiple meals throughout the week.

7. Prep Vegetables in Advance:
   - Wash, chop, and portion vegetables ahead of time. They can be used in salads, stir-fries, or as snacks.
8. Portion Control:
   - Use measuring tools to ensure accurate portion sizes. This minimizes overeating and aids in calorie control.
9. Utilize Freezer-Friendly Options:
   - Prepare and freeze meals that can be easily reheated, especially for days when you have less time to cook.
10. Mix and Match Components:
    - Prepare individual components (e.g., roasted vegetables, grilled chicken) that can be mixed and matched to create various meals.
11. Prep Breakfasts:
    - Consider prepping breakfast options like overnight oats, smoothie ingredients, or egg

muffins for a quick and healthy start to the day.

12. Prep Snacks:
    - Have healthy snacks like cut-up veggies, hummus, or portioned nuts readily available to curb midday cravings.

13. Label and Date:
    - Label containers with the date of preparation and any reheating instructions. This ensures you use meals before they lose freshness.

14. Stay Organized:
    - Keep your kitchen organized to streamline the prep process. Arrange ingredients and tools in a way that makes the workflow efficient.

15. Experiment with Flavors:
    - Use a variety of herbs, spices, and marinades to add flavor to your meals. This prevents monotony and keeps your taste buds satisfied.

16. Prep Grains and Pasta:
    - Cook a batch of whole grains (quinoa, brown rice) or whole

wheat pasta to use as a base for
different meals.

17. Consider Crockpot or Instant Pot Meals:
    - Utilize slow cookers or instant pots for hands-off cooking of stews, soups, or one-pot meals.
18. Mindful Reheating:
    - When reheating, use methods that preserve the nutritional value of your meals. To keep vegetables crunchy, don't overcook them.
19. Make it Enjoyable:
    - Choose recipes you enjoy eating. This makes it more likely that you'll stick to your meal prepping routine.
20. Stay Consistent:
    - Consistency is key. Stick to your meal prepping routine, and it will become a valuable habit for maintaining a healthy lifestyle.

Meal prepping can be as simple or as elaborate as you like. Experiment with different approaches to find a routine that works best for your schedule and preferences.

SEEKING PROFESSIONAL GUIDANCE

Seeking professional guidance is a commendable step toward achieving your health and wellness goals. Here are some professionals you might consider consulting:

1. Registered Dietitian (RD) or Nutritionist:
   - A registered dietitian can provide personalized nutrition advice based on your health goals, dietary preferences, and any medical conditions.
2. Certified Personal Trainer:
   - If you're looking to improve your fitness level or develop a workout routine, a certified personal trainer can create a tailored exercise plan.
3. Health Coach:
   - A health coach can assist you in setting and achieving health-related goals, offering support

and guidance in areas like nutrition, exercise, and stress management.

4. Primary Care Physician:
    - Your primary care doctor can provide a comprehensive health assessment, address any underlying medical concerns, and guide you toward appropriate specialists.
5. Endocrinologist:
    - For issues related to hormonal changes, especially during menopause, consulting an endocrinologist may be beneficial.
6. Gynecologist:
    - Women over 40 may benefit from consulting a gynecologist for specific health concerns related to menopause, reproductive health, and overall well-being.
7. Psychologist or Counselor:
    - A mental health professional can support you in managing stress, anxiety, or any emotional factors influencing your health journey.
8. Physical Therapist:

- If you have specific physical concerns or injuries, a physical therapist can provide exercises and strategies for improvement.

9. Sleep Specialist:
    - If you're struggling with sleep issues, a sleep specialist can assess your sleep patterns and provide guidance on improving sleep quality.

10. Allergist or Immunologist:
    - If you suspect food allergies or sensitivities, consulting an allergist or immunologist can help identify and manage these issues.

11. Chiropractor or Physiotherapist:
    - For musculoskeletal concerns or chronic pain, a chiropractor or physiotherapist can offer assessment and treatment.

12. Wellness Program:
    - Some workplaces or community centers offer wellness programs that include guidance from nutritionists, fitness trainers, and mental health professionals.

13. Pharmacist:

- ○ Your pharmacist can provide information about medications and supplements, including potential interactions and side effects.
14. Online Platforms:
    - ○ Consider reputable online platforms that connect you with virtual health professionals, offering consultations and personalized guidance.
15. Genetic Counselor:
    - ○ If you're interested in understanding your genetic predispositions related to health, a genetic counselor can provide insights and recommendations.

Remember to communicate openly with these professionals about your goals, concerns, and any existing health conditions. Their expertise can provide you with a well-rounded and individualized approach to achieving a healthier lifestyle.

SUSTAINABLE LIFESTYLE CHANGES

Creating sustainable lifestyle changes involves making adjustments that you can maintain over the long term. Here are some tips for adopting and maintaining a healthier lifestyle:

1. Start Small:
    - Begin with manageable changes. It can be daunting to attempt a complete lifestyle makeover all at once. Small, consistent steps are more sustainable.
2. Set Realistic Goals:
    - Define achievable, specific, and realistic goals. Divide more ambitious objectives into smaller, more doable tasks.
3. Focus on Habits, Not Diets:
    - Shift your focus from short-term diets to long-term habits. Aim for changes that become a natural part of your daily routine.
4. Build Gradually:
    - Add new habits gradually. For example, if you're working on

nutrition, focus on adding more vegetables to your meals before eliminating certain foods.

5. Make It Enjoyable:
   - Choose activities and foods you enjoy. Joy in the process increases the likelihood that you will persevere.
6. Involve Others:
   - Share your goals with friends or family and encourage them to join you. Having a support system can make the journey more enjoyable and sustainable.
7. Prioritize Sleep:
   - Ensure you're getting sufficient, quality sleep. Sleep is crucial for overall well-being and can impact your ability to make healthy choices.
8. Practice Mindful Eating:
   - Pay attention to your body's hunger and fullness cues. Consume food only when you're hungry and quit when you're full.
9. Learn from Setbacks:
   - Recognize that obstacles are a typical part of any journey.

Instead of dwelling on them, learn from them and adjust your approach as needed.

10. Create a Routine:
    - Establish a daily routine that includes time for healthy habits. Consistency fosters habit formation.
11. Stay Hydrated:
    - Drink enough water throughout the day. Proper hydration supports overall health and can positively impact your energy levels.
12. Incorporate Physical Activity You Enjoy:
    - Find forms of exercise that you genuinely enjoy. You're more likely to persevere if you do this.
13. Plan Your Meals:
    - Plan and prepare your meals in advance. As a result, there is a decreased chance of depending on junk food.
14. Explore New Foods:
    - Expand your palate by trying new, nutritious foods. This can add variety to your diet and make it more interesting.

15. Mindful Stress Management:
    - Include stress-reduction methods in your routine, such as yoga, deep breathing, or meditation.
16. Celebrate Achievements:
    - Celebrate your successes, whether big or small. Reward and acknowledge yourself when you accomplish goals.
17. Keep Learning:
    - Stay informed about nutrition, fitness, and overall wellness. The more you know, the better equipped you are to make informed choices.
18. Be Patient:
    - Sustainable changes take time. Treat yourself with kindness and acknowledge the strides you make in the process.
19. Evaluate and Adjust:
    - Periodically assess your habits and make adjustments as needed. Your needs and circumstances may change over time.
20. Enjoy the Journey:

- o Embrace the process of creating a healthier lifestyle. The journey itself is valuable, and every positive choice contributes to your well-being.

Remember, sustainability is about creating a lifestyle that aligns with your values and brings you joy. It's not about perfection but about progress and making choices that support your long-term health and happiness.

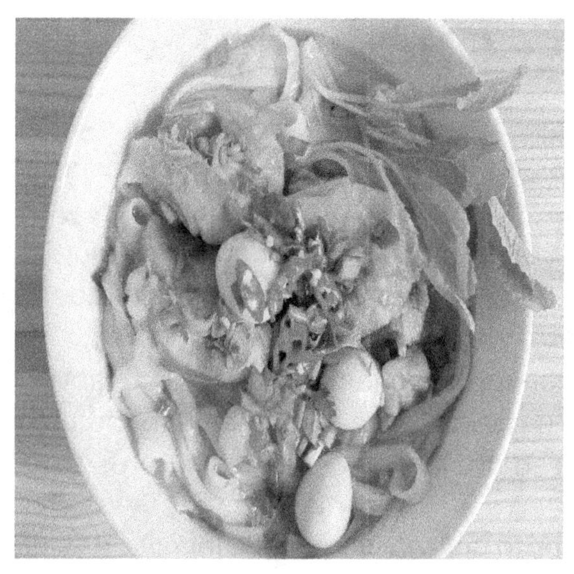

CONCLUSION

In conclusion, embarking on a journey towards a healthier and more sustainable lifestyle involves a thoughtful combination of mindful choices, gradual changes, and a commitment to long-term well-being. By adopting small, achievable steps and incorporating enjoyable habits, you can create a sustainable foundation for improved health.

Remember to set realistic goals, involve a support system, prioritize sleep, and stay hydrated. Make choices that bring you joy, whether in physical activities or the foods you consume. Mindful eating, stress management, and regular evaluations of your habits contribute to a holistic approach.

Celebrate your achievements, no matter how small, and acknowledge that setbacks are opportunities for growth. Embrace the learning process and continuously strive for progress rather than perfection.

As you navigate this journey, keep in mind that a sustainable lifestyle is a personalized and evolving path. Enjoy the process, cherish the positive changes you make, and let the journey towards a healthier you be fulfilling and rewarding.

RECAP OF KEY PRINCIPLES

Here's a recap of key principles for adopting a healthier and more sustainable lifestyle:

1. Start Small and Gradual:
    - Begin with manageable changes and gradually build on them to make the transition more sustainable.
2. Set Realistic and Achievable Goals:
    - Define specific, realistic goals that you can realistically achieve over time.
3. Focus on Habits, Not Diets:
    - Shift your focus from short-term diets to long-term, sustainable habits for lasting health benefits.
4. Enjoyable Choices:

- Choose activities, exercises, and foods that bring you joy to enhance long-term adherence.

5. Involve a Support System:
    - Share your goals with friends or family to create a support system that encourages and motivates you.
6. Prioritize Quality Sleep:
    - Ensure you get sufficient, quality sleep as it plays a crucial role in overall well-being.
7. Mindful Eating:
    - Pay attention to your body's signals of hunger and fullness when you eat mindfully.
8. Learn from Setbacks:
    - Treat setbacks as learning opportunities and adjust your approach accordingly.
9. Establish a Routine:
    - Create a daily routine that incorporates time for healthy habits, promoting consistency.
10. Stay Hydrated:
    - Drink enough water throughout the day to support overall health and energy levels.

11. Incorporate Enjoyable Physical Activity:
    ○ Choose forms of exercise that you genuinely enjoy to make it a sustainable part of your routine.
12. Plan and Prepare Meals:
    ○ Make meal plans and prepare your food ahead of time to stay away from unhealthy convenience foods.
13. Explore New Nutritious Foods:
    ○ Experiment with new, nutritious foods to add variety and interest to your diet.
14. Mindful Stress Management:
    ○ Incorporate stress management techniques such as meditation, deep breathing, or yoga.
15. Celebrate Achievements:
    ○ Acknowledge and reward yourself for reaching milestones, no matter how small.
16. Continuous Learning:
    ○ Stay informed about nutrition, fitness, and overall wellness to make informed choices.
17. Patience and Progress:

- Treat yourself with kindness and acknowledge the strides you make in the process.

18. Evaluate and Adjust:
    - Periodically assess your habits and make adjustments based on changing needs and circumstances.

19. Enjoy the Journey:
    - Embrace the process of creating a healthier lifestyle, recognizing that the journey itself is valuable.

20. Strive for Progress, Not Perfection:
    - Aim for continuous improvement rather than perfection. Progress over time is the key to lasting change.

Keep in mind that every wise decision you make enhances your general wellbeing. It's the collective impact of these choices that leads to a healthier and more fulfilling lifestyle.

ENCOURAGEMENT FOR LONG-TERM HEALTH

Congratulations on taking steps toward long-term health! Recall that this is a marathon, not a sprint, on this journey. Here are some words of motivation to keep you going:

1. Celebrate Every Step:
    - Celebrate and acknowledge your accomplishments, no matter how small. Every positive choice contributes to your overall well-being.
2. Embrace Consistency:
    - Sustainable change comes from consistent efforts. Focus on making healthy choices a regular part of your routine.
3. Learn and Grow:
    - View setbacks as opportunities to learn and grow. Use them to refine your approach and continue progressing.
4. Patience is Key:
    - Be patient with yourself. Sustainable health is a journey

that takes time. Take pleasure in the transformation into a healthier version of yourself.

5. Enjoy the Journey:
   - Find joy in the changes you're making. Whether it's trying new recipes, discovering new physical activities, or feeling increased energy, savor the positive aspects of your journey.
6. Listen to Your Body:
   - Pay attention to how your body responds to different habits. It's a powerful guide for understanding what works best for you.
7. Adapt and Adjust:
   - Your journey may evolve, and that's perfectly okay. Adapt your approach as needed, keeping your long-term health goals in mind.
8. Stay Connected:
   - Talk about your journey with loved ones, close friends, or a community of support. Connection and encouragement can be powerful motivators.
9. Prioritize Self-Care:

- Remember that taking care of your health is an act of self-love. Prioritize self-care and make choices that nurture your well-being.

10. Visualize Your Success:
    - Envision the healthy, vibrant version of yourself that you're working towards. This idea in your mind can be a strong incentive.
11. Be Proud of Your Efforts:
    - You've already taken important steps towards better health. Be proud of the positive choices you're making for yourself.
12. Reflect on Progress:
    - Regularly reflect on how far you've come. It's a great way to stay motivated and appreciate the positive changes in your life.
13. Celebrate Non-Scale Victories:
    - Not all victories are measured on a scale. Celebrate improvements in energy, mood, sleep quality, and overall well-being.
14. Inspire Others:

- ○ Others may be motivated to prioritize their health by your journey. Share your experiences and encourage those around you.
15. Focus on Wellness, Not Perfection:
    - ○ Aim for overall wellness rather than perfection. It's the combination of positive habits that leads to lasting health.

Remember, each day is an opportunity to make choices that contribute to your long-term well-being. Stay committed, stay positive, and enjoy the ongoing journey towards a healthier and happier you!

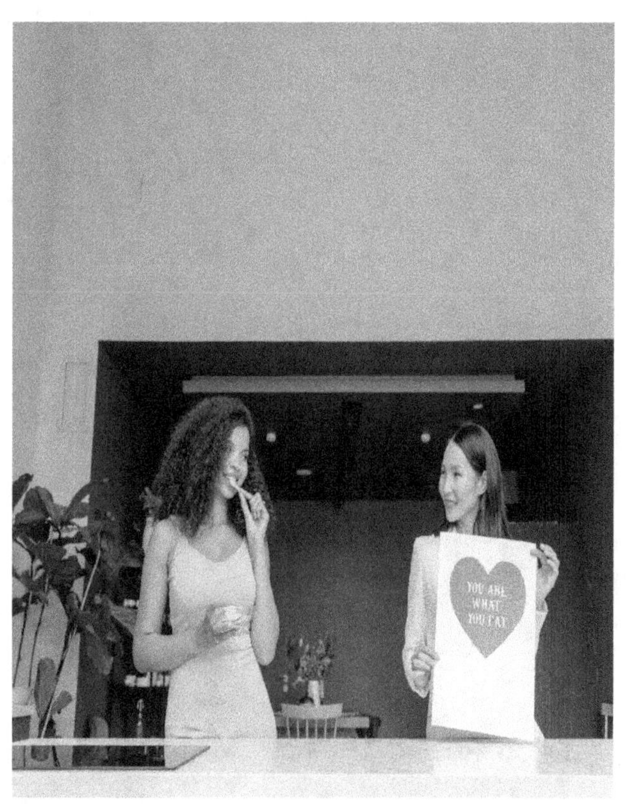

YOU ARE
WHAT
YOU EAT

www.ingramcontent.com/pod-product-compliance
Lightning Source LLC
Chambersburg PA
CBHW070938260726
48661CB00003B/1032